# AIDS

## IMPACT ON PUBLIC POLICY

An International Forum: Policy, Politics, and AIDS

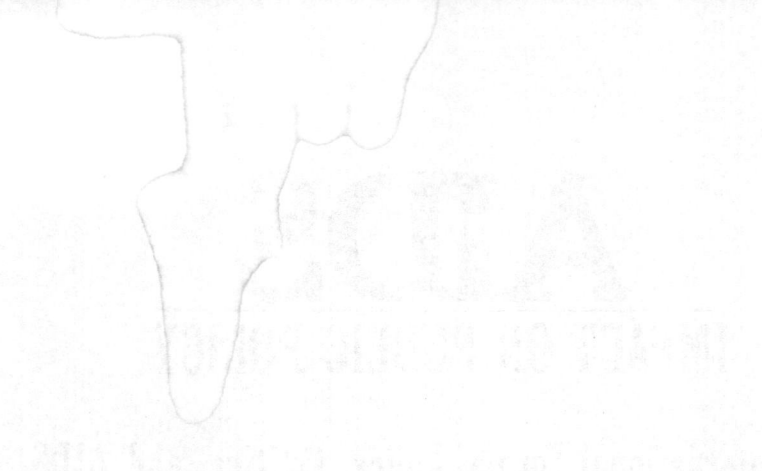

# AIDS
## IMPACT ON PUBLIC POLICY

An International Forum: Policy, Politics, and AIDS

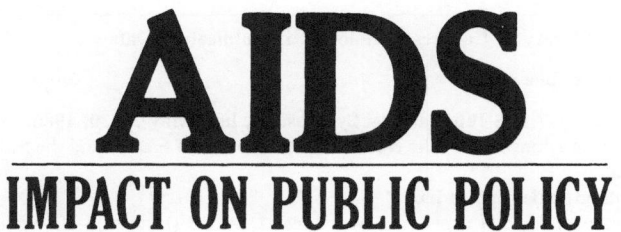

Edited by
### Robert F. Hummel
### William F. Leavy
### Michael Rampolla
and
### Sherry Chorost
*New York State Department of Health*
*Albany, New York*

PLENUM PRESS • NEW YORK AND LONDON

Library of Congress Cataloging in Publication Data

AIDS, impact on public policy.

Proceedings of the AIDS International Symposium, held May 28–30, 1986, in New York, N.Y., and co-sponsored by the New York State Dept. of Health and the Milbank Memorial Fund.
Includes bibliographies and index.
1. AIDS (Disease) — Social aspects — Congresses. 2. AIDS (Disease) — Government policy — Congresses. 3. AIDS (Disease) — Prevention — Congresses. I. Hummel, Robert F. II. AIDS International Symposium (1986: New York, N.Y.) III. New York (State) Dept. of Health. IV. Milbank Memorial Fund. [DNLM: 1. Acquired Immunodeficiency Syndrome — prevention & control — congresses. 2. International Cooperation — congresses. 3. Public Policy — congresses. WD 308 A28834 1986]
RA644.A25A363   1986                     362.1'96997'92                     86-30516
ISBN-13: 978-1-4615-9491-8        e-ISBN-13: 978-1-4615-9489-5
DOI: 10.1007/ 978-1-4615-9489-5

Proceedings of a conference cosponsored by the New York
State Department of Health and the Milbank Memorial Fund,
held May 28–30, 1986, in New York, New York

© 1986 Plenum Press, New York
**Softcover reprint of the hardcover 1st edition 1986**
A Division of Plenum Publishing Corporation
233 Spring Street, New York, N.Y. 10013

This conference was cosponsored by the New York State Department of Health and the Milbank Memorial Fund.

DAVID AXELROD, M.D.
Commissioner
New York State Department of Health

SIDNEY LEE, M.D., Dr. P.H.
President
Milbank Memorial Fund

MEL ROSEN, C.S.W.
Director
AIDS Institute

GOVERNOR MARIO CUOMO
Governor, New York

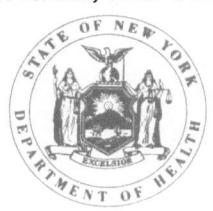

## PREFACE

Acquired Immune Deficiency Syndrome continues to be a major
concern of the research and health care communities as well as the
dominant public health issue in the news media. In the early years
of the epidemic, attention was appropriately focused on
characterizing the epidemiology of the disease in order to define
the nature and extent of this new threat. However, as the disease
affected the lives of ever increasing thousands of individuals and
spread to almost every country, its ramifications were felt at every
level of society. In addition to medical and research issues,
profound social, economic and moral dilemmas have arisen. The
implications which AIDS has on public policy continue to unfold.

Recognizing the value of assembling those who were involved with
AIDS on a national and international level, New York State through
its Health Department brought together social scientists,
researchers, clinicians, educators, community leaders, government
officials and public policy analysts to explore and discuss major
AIDS public policy issues at the AIDS International Symposium.

This volume includes both the major papers presented as well as
the discussions among the panel members which followed the
presentations. Clearly, the conference demonstrated the
international nature of AIDS as a public health and public policy
problem. Evident also is that the devleopment of public policy
properly begins as a dialogue, both at the interpersonal and
international levels, and that the process is never complete,
particularly when it concerns the type of threat that AIDS presents
to the world community.

The editors wish to thank Governor Mario Cuomo and Commissioner
David Axelrod. Without their vision and support, the conference
would never have become a reality. In addition, recognition is
given to the work of Ms. Rose Marie Anatriello whose skill and
dedication made this volume possible.

Robert F. Hummel
William Leavy
Michael Rampolla
Sherry Chorost

# CONTENTS

WELCOMING REMARKS


David Axelrod, M.D.[1],
David Sencer, M.D., M.P.H.[2], and
Edward Koch[3]


### Dr. Axelrod

I would like to welcome you on behalf of the Governor of the
State of New York, Mario Cuomo, to what I hope will be an
informative and evocative forum on a pressing public health issue.
I have a certain degree of mixed feeling about welcoming you to a
conference, the subject of which has been such an enormous problem
to all of those who are here and certainly to those of us in New
York State, especially those who represent some of the major urban
areas where AIDS has been a continuing problem.  I'm delighted that
this conference has attracted individuals from a broad spectrum of
the world community, because AIDS is not only a problem for this
state or the nation, but rather for people everywhere on this planet.

I'd like to publicly acknowledge, at this point, the enormous
help that we've had from the Milbank Memorial Fund in developing the
program.  Without the assistance of the Milbank Memorial Fund we
could not have gathered a faculty of this diversity and excellence.

I need not comment on the appropriateness of the venue of this
conference.  Certainly there isn't a soul in this room who doesn't
recognize that AIDS has hit this city and state particularly hard.
Almost 7,000 New Yorkers have been stricken with the disease and
over half of them have died.  AIDS is today the leading cause of
death among young men in this state.  The rate at which new cases
are being discovered in New York State continues to rise.  We
believe, on the basis of current epidemiologic evidence, that
hundreds of thousands of New Yorkers have been exposed to the virus
that is associated with AIDS.  The 417 new cases reported in the 36
days ending April 21, sustain this prediction.

The cost of the AIDS epidemic in suffering, premature death, and
economics, is beyond measure.  In this state the typical AIDS
patient will spend a total of three weeks in-hospital during the

---

[1] Commissioner, New York State Department of Health
[2] Director, Management Science for Health   [3]  Mayor, City of
New York

course of his or her disease, and during that time he or she will be responsible for medical costs of between $50,000 and $100,000. Last year in this state the average monthly total of AIDS patients admitted to the hospital was 473, and the admission rate increased at about three and a half percent per month. This year, the State of New York, in an effort to deal with the problem of providing adequate communal services to those in the AIDS population, will designate at least 15 centers as AIDS treatment centers. These centers, located in hospitals, will care for a majority of the state's AIDS patients who require in-patient services. In recognition of the high costs that we have found associated with the care of these patients, and the intensity of the care that is required, these hospitals' reimbursements are being increased by the state to ensure that the costs are being met by the reimbursement system.

We estimate that there are some 200,000 IV drug users in New York City alone who are active and represent a potential threat to the continuing number of cases that are being reported. We are launching a community oriented, bilingual educational campaign to inform the IV drug user population about the risks of AIDS both to themselves and to those they love. Motivating this population represents an enormous challenge to the educational component of our AIDS program. Until a vaccine or another effective means of treating or preventing AIDS is found, our goal must be to break the chain of virus transmission. That means that we must communicate repeatedly and clearly and effectively with at-risk populations and convince them to change those practices which place them at risk to their lives and to the lives of those they hold most dear. There's probably no arena in which there has been greater controversy than in the development of public policies for community health, as opposed to individual rights.

The devastating effect of AIDS; its severity, its impact on at-risk populations, the fears that it has generated in the general populace, have created an enormous challenge to our political structure, to medical science and to our health institutions and social agencies. Our public/private health partnership is being stressed to an uncommon degree. To government, AIDS represents a test of the social covenant to protect the health and safety of all of the citizenry. To medical science, AIDS heralds the onset of vastly more complex viral diseases than any we have encountered before. To the human species, AIDS is the latest chapter in mankind's eternal struggle with infectious organisms, a struggle which some had thought was over. Through this forum, we hope to contribute to a larger understanding of the numerous social, medical and economic issues surrounding AIDS, and of the role of governments around the world in responding to them. My expectation is that there will be controversy, there will be confrontation, and out of this confrontation will come recommendations for changes in existing public policy, and the initiation of new efforts for the prevention of the spread of this disease. I hope that the exchanges will be frank and I assume that they will be rewarding to all of those who are here. I thank you very much for being here and for participating in this very, very critical conference.

The title of this conference is "AIDS: Impact on Public Policy." The title presents the problem. Should we not be talking about the impact of public policy upon AIDS? Should not public policy be proactive rather than reactive?

A reactive public policy says, "Exclude from schools. Deny employment. Discriminate." A proactive public policy should find methods to prevent transmission of HIV, based on ethical science rather than expediency and emotion.

Transmission of HIV is overwhelmingly the result of human behavior, but the small successes that have been achieved in preventing transmission have been in other areas where traditional public policy approaches have been used - - research and regulation. Research has developed a method of screening blood for evidence of infection and regulation has implemented the use of the test. The same is true for the inactivation of the virus in plasma.

Can the existing public policies contribute further to preventing the spread of infection in this country? To what extent can public policies bend in stemming the epidemic of drug abuse? Proactive public policy has stimulated and supported attempts at education as a method of behavior modification, although many will say too little and too late. But there are reactive public policies that prevent some individuals from modifying their behavior even when they want to. Let me mention just one.

The mayor will give you an official welcome, but let me welcome you to a city that has an estimated 250,000 desperately ill people. Ill because they are addicted to heroin and use needles and syringes to "treat" themselves. Public policy (FDA Regulations) limit treatment to clinics that provide not only medical supervision, but a complete array of services -- laboratory screening, social and rehabilitative services. The most widely used method of treatment, methadone maintenance, is available to only 22,000 of the 250,000 addicted individuals in New York City. And there are waiting lists.

Public policy limits treatment by its inadequate funding. Public policy bodies object to the placement of treatment centers in their neighborhoods. (The only thing worse than a shelter for the homeless, is a drug treatment center!)

The Special Prosecuter of Substance Abuse in New York City characterized the life of an addict as: Two hours wanting treatment, but the next six hours trying to find the money to buy his next needed heroin.

Shouldn't public policy recognize that those two hours are windows to possible change? Shouldn't methadone become as available as any prescription drug? Each time an addicted person swallows methadone rather than injecting heroin there is one less chance of transmission of HIV. Most times that methadone replaces heroin, a crime is prevented. Each consecutive time that methadone replaces heroin there is hope for the ill.

I know of no other widely used and understood drug that is withheld by Federal Regulation, unless an entire battery of services is available. By allowing this public policy to remain unchallenged, we not only perpetuate heroin addiction, but we promote the spread of HIV. The Hippocratic Oath instructs us to do no harm. By not demanding that addiction be approached as an illness rather than a crime we are doing harm. We harm the addict, his sexual partner and their potential progeny.

I overheard a conversation between Drs. Axelrod and Lee before the meeting in which they hoped that this conference would stimulate discussion and controversy. I hope that I have helped them meet this goal and that discussion of the ethical dilemmas of drug abuse and treatment will lead to a change in public policy.

Thank you.


## Mayor Koch

What I would like to do, instead of bringing "Coals to Newcastle" and exhibit my knowledge of the facts of which you have far greater knowledge, I would like to make a short statement.

The City of New York is proud of what we have done in responding to a catastrophe. I can tell you that the person that we're proudest of, who has led the fight here in the city, regrettably no longer with us, is Dr. David Sencer who was our health commissioner and who did an extraordinary job. What we are proud of - at least what I'm terribly proud of - relates to our response to the AIDS patients, those in need, and also leading the fight to make certain that children who have AIDS could go to school. There was a case which went on endlessly, went on a couple of months. The leading witness was Dr. Sencer before a very hostile judge. We know he was hostile by the comments that he made in the course of the trial. But the proofs submitted by the city were so overwhelming on the subject that his decision, which went on endlessly too, came out in favor of the city. And children in the City of New York, who have AIDS, go to school. It's a landmark decision and I suspect that other jurisdictions are using it as well. What I believe the federal government ought to be doing that it is not doing, amongst other things, and I'll leave the other things to you, is to take over the total cost of the care of patients in the same way that it does for those that need renal dialysis and places them immediately under SSI, a form of social security medicare benefits. They should do the same for those suffering from AIDS, because not to do that is causing havoc financially in the municipal hospital sector and equally, or more so, in the voluntary hospital sector. Firstly, the hospitals are becoming terribly burdened with treating this single disease. Secondly, the payment made to the various hospitals does not correspond to the cost. It's about $200.00 short on the average, each day of patient care, and that then becomes borne by the locality. If it's a municipal hospital it comes out of our city treasury, if it's a voluntary hospital it comes out of their endowment and their funds that they raise through charitable drives. That's wrong. It should be a total takeover by the federal government. (A brief period of questions and answers followed, but have not been reproduced)

4

Keynote Address:  Heterosexual Transmission:  Fear or Reality

Nathan Clumeck, M.D., Ph.D.
Associate Professor of Infectious Diseases
Free University of Brussels, Belgium

KEYNOTE ADDRESS:    HETEROSEXUAL TRANSMISSION: FEAR OR REALITY

Nathan Clumeck, M.D., Ph.D.

Associate Professor of Infectious Diseases
Free University of Brussels, Belgium

Mr. Chairman, ladies and gentlemen, as you know, to date 18 western countries are experiencing tremendous problems among male homosexuals, bisexuals and IV drug users.  So far, the epidemic is uncontrolled and no vaccine or chemical therapeutic agents have prevented infection or reduced infectivity.  One of our major concerns is preventing the spread of AIDS into the general population.  In this view, the extreme attitudes which consist either of dogmatically negating bidirectional transmission of the AIDS virus, or of hysterical concern over serious limitations of a civil right, need to be balanced by an accurate perception of risk to heterosexuals.  From this perspective, the question is, will western civilization survive an AIDS epidemic?

Assuming that the number of AIDS cases is doubling every six months, there would be no uninfected American left in 1993.  This view is aimed at provoking panic and supporting claims for quarantine measures.  Fortunately, heterosexual spread, while existing, is far less alarming. As you know, heterosexual spread is a major concern in African countries.  In Brussels, where we see many African people, the number of cases since 1982 has been increasing.  We saw our first homosexual patient in Belgium in the middle of 1984 and all the other cases were heterosexual people.

If we want to evaluate the risk of heterosexual transmission, various factors have to be considered.  First, the prevalence of AIDS virus infection in the heterosexual community.  Second, the efficiency of transmission.  Third, promiscuity of a population. Since there are sharp discrepancies between the spreading of AIDS in western countries and African countries we have also to consider yet unidentified behavioral or biological factors.

What about the prevalence of the AIDS virus in the general community?  In order to evaluate this prevalence we disposed of results of blood donor studies, which clearly showed that in western countries the prevalence is very low in the general population in contrast with four to eighteen percent of seroprevalence among the heterosexual population in most central African countries. However, these numbers are related to the general population, and if we are talking about a sexually transmitted disease we have to look for a high risk group in the heterosexual population namely, female prostitutes. First, in central African countries, there is no doubt that female prostitutes are a high risk group for HIV infection since the prevalence varies between 30 percent and more than 80 percent in the groups studied. In western countries the situation is quite different, although the studies are limited to small groups. In London and Paris studies, zero percent prevalence was found. In West Germany, there is controversy about the rate of prevalence among prostitutes. A number between 1 and 20 percent is cited. In the United States 40 percent among the prostitutes in Miami, five percent in Seattle.

In western countries it is found that most seropositive prostitutes admit to IV drug use and since these prostitutes can constitute a reservoir of the AIDS virus, it's important to evaluate the numbers of seropositives among the IV drug users, but also among the heterosexual contacts of persons at high risk, or among the person at no known risk which clearly delineates the people who have heterosexual promiscuity. Following a mode of calculation published by Syvac and Wanther in the New England Journal of Medicine, assuming that you multiply by 300 the number of AIDS cases living, you obtain a rough estimation of the number of seropositive. We can then estimate that in 1985 more than 348,000 people were seropositive, and this number doubled in less than one year. This is a rough estimation of the potential heterosexual reservoir in the American general population.

The second point is the efficiency of the transmission of HIV for heterosexual activity? I think that there are no doubts that evidence exists of bidirectional transmission of the AIDS virus, but also that female to male sexual transmission could be less efficient than transmission from male to female. Since the beginning of the epidemic there was evidence from studies of female sexual partners of hemophiliacs and IV drug users that the male was able to transmit the AIDS virus to his female partner. I think it's important to note that there is no need of receptive anal intercourse. And normal sexual activity could transmit the virus. What's the efficiency of this transmission?

In studies of hemophiliac groups, the number of seropositives among spouse or sexual partners varies between nine and 71 percent. That's clearly the evidence. In spite of the fact that males can easily transmit the virus, we need also to determine other factors, such as the frequency of sexual activity and other factors yet unknown. For the male IV drug user a very interesting study has just been published which shows that in couples of IV drug users where the male partner was positive, and the female was not an IV drug user, only eight percent of seropositivity was noted among the partners. When both were IV drug abusers 58 percent were positive. This is a clear indication about the AIDS virus transmission. Injecting the virus directly into the blood stream is efficient and appears more efficient than heterosexual activity. However, studies from Australia on cryopreserved semen of a carrier of HIV, note in a small study, that 50 percent of recipients were positive after artificial insemination. One could then assume that the efficiency of transmission is probably also linked to sexual activity and its frequency.

We have a good indication of such hypothesis from African studies. In the group of premarital adolescents from Rwanda, girls between 16 to 18 before marriage, zero percent seropositivity was found. Among the group of married women from various studies from Kinshasa in Zaire, five to 10 percent seroprevalence was found. Among the group of highly promiscuous women - so-called "free women" in Africa - their prevalence varied between 30 to 80 percent. So the AIDS virus is efficiently transmitted from male to female, but it is necessary to have promiscuous activity in order to get the virus.

Now what about the female to male sexual transmission. This point is highly controversial. HIV has been isolated from vaginal and cervical secretions. So the potential exists for such transmission from normal vaginal intercourse. Evidence of female to male sexual transmission exists in the epidemiology of the African epidemic, from a study from the Walter Reed Army study of American soldiers, from CDC studies of men of unknown risk, and also from individual case reports recently published. Among the men with AIDS studied by Redfield, it was found that 37 percent of patients with AIDS admitted to no risk factor, excepting either heterosexual contact with partners, female partners who developed AIDS, or multiple heterosexual partners, and all reported sexual contacts with female prostitutes. This is the first study which showed that female to male transmission could occur in western countries.

What about the occurrence of female to male transmission in Africa? First the demography of AIDS in equatorial Africa strongly suggests that this transmission is bidirectional. The male to female ratio is nearly one. All the people with AIDS are young to middle-aged men and women, or children aged less than five years. Two-thirds of the female and one-third of the males are single. And when risk factors were examined among this population, heterosexual promiscuity was the only risk factor found among patients, or among their sexual partners.

In a study performed in Rwanda, Van de Perre found that male customers of prostitutes presented a 30 percent seroprevalence in comparison with male controls without contact with prostitutes. And this difference between the male customers and the male controls was highly significant. In a case controlled study of African patients with AIDS in comparison with age and socially matched group, we found that the patient with AIDS admitted regular contacts with prostitutes in 81 percent in comparison with 34 percent of controls. And this was highly significant. The patient with AIDS had more partners, a mean of 32 per year, in comparison with three in the control group. In addition, when we looked for the relative risk of seroprevalence among the male customer of prostitutes, we found that increasing the numbers of sexual partners showed a significant increase of the seroprevalence among people who had contact with prostitutes.

I think it's most important to note that these contacts were mainly penis/vaginal contacts as found by questioning the prostitutes. And this study has just been confirmed very recently by other studies in Kinshasa. However, we have to also account for additional factors or co-factors which could explain why the spread of AIDS is so explosive in central Africa. Factors to consider are: the existence of inflammatory disease of genitourinary tract among patients, behavioral differences such as sexual contact during menses, trauma during sex, anal intercourse, and most important to

9

me are co-infections with other pathogens, other sexually transmitted diseases and an altered immunological status at the time of infection.

However, what is the rate of spread of the HIV virus into the general population? If we look now from studies performed by Desmyter in Brussels and Piot in Antwerp who looked at married women from Kinshasa and stored serum from 1970, the seroprevalence confirmed by ELISA, Western blot, immunofluorescence was 0.25 percent which is actually the seroprevalence in our general population in western countries. Ten years later this seroprevalence was three percent. So during a 10-year period among the general population, assuming nonpromiscuous women, the increase of the seroprevalence was 10-fold for 10 years. The same increase was observed among pregnant women from Kenya, zero percent seroprevalence in 1981 and five years later two percent seroprevalence. The findings are quite different among the female prostitutes as a group. In 1981 there was four percent seroprevalence in Kenyan prostitutes. And five years later about 60 percent seroprevalence. Most interesting, the same increase was found among heterosexual men from Kenya, with STD, zero percent seroprevalence in 1981 and four years later 14 percent prevalence. This has to be compared with the increase of the seropositivity among the San Francisco cohort of homosexuals or bisexuals. One can assume from these studies that the potential exists for heterosexual transmission into the general population through heterosexual activity.

However, some people think that heterosexual activity is not an important means of transmission of the AIDS virus, and criticism has been expressed of these studies. The first criticism is that female to male transmission is not well documented, and is based on the assumption that prostitutes are a source of the virus. The second criticism is the lack of control groups in western countries between people that used and did not use prostitutes in related HIV antibody stages. The third criticism centers on whether the prostitutes are exposed to a marker or some other risk factors such as receiving intramuscular injection with dirty needles for transmittal of STD's.

We have to look for future heterosexual spread of AIDS in western countries. Two points of view exist, the optimistic and the pessimistic one.

The optimistic point of view assumes that the percentage of heterosexual patients will remain stable, because it has been stable since 1981. In fact, it has increased since 1981. The percentage is stable, but the numbers of cases have increased while the percentage stayed the same. The second point is that female to male transmission will occur less easily than male to female. The third point is that the situation in Africa is due to unrecognized factors not likely to occur in northern countries. The last point is that a mass education campaign will be successful in changing practices of promiscuous heterosexuals.

The pessimistic point of view is that the pool of infected heterosexual males and females will increase, since bisexual and IV drug abusers are a bridge to heterosexual people, that most female IV drug users practice prostitution, and most important due to the low prevalence, at present, of the virus in the general population, the perception of the risk of HIV infection is not perceived by promiscuous heterosexuals who won't change their sexual lifestyle.

What can be proposed as a strategic tool for controlling heterosexual spread? First, since the numbers of seropositives among the heterosexual community is low in comparison with positivity in homosexuals, or bisexuals, or IV drug users, individual education and counseling of infected heterosexuals could be effective. Tracking, testing, interviewing and counseling the contact is very important. The educational campaign must be centralized and directed towards potential sexually active high school students. And the last point, screening for the AIDS virus in people at risk early in pregnancy or premaritally. We have performed such studies in Brussels. The experience of our hospital is very preliminary, but could be indicative of such experience. We required an informed consent of the pregnant woman and we assured the confidentiality of the results. We studied the women assumed to be at risk in Brussels. That means women originating or living in sub-Saharan countries, IV drug abusers and prostitutes. And we performed the ELISA test confirmed by Western blot. During a six month period more than 600 pregnant women registered. Approximately nine percent of these were in risk groups and the results of seroprevalence studies of these high risk women showed that 11 percent of them were HIV seropositive. Five women were from central Africa, two were IV drug users. The most important point is that all were healthy without any sign or symptom of HIV infection. These women delivered normal children and delivery occurred with routine procedures. We tested, examined and counseled the spouses or sexual partners of these women, and in all cases the men were highly promiscuous. We educated about the nature of HIV infection and its transmission, and we discussed further birth control. We also arranged psychosocial support which was very important in these cases.

In conclusion, in western countries there is no concern about the epidemic spreading of AIDS virus into the general population. However, the possibility exists of outward spread of AIDS to non-homosexual, bisexual and to non-drug users. We have to prevent that now. And this prevention constitutes a tremendous challenge and any risk reduction therefore has to begin early, if we want to be successful. Thank you very much.

Session A:  Public Health and Private Rights:  Health, Social
and Ethical Perspectives

<u>Participants</u>

<u>Speakers</u>

Harvey Fineberg, M.D., Ph.D.
Dean, Harvard School of Public Health

Thomas Vernon, M.D.
Executive Director, Colorado Department of Health

<u>Panelists</u>

Ronald Bayer, Ph.D.
Associate for Policy Studies, The Hastings Center

James Childress, Ph.D.
Kyle Professor of Religious Studies and
Professor of Medical Education, University of Virginia

Dean Echenberg, M.D., Ph.D.
Director, Bureau of Communicable Disease Control, Department
of Public Health, City and County of San Francisco

Michael Adler, M.D.
Chairman, Department of Genito-urinary Medicine, Middlesex
Hospital Medical School, London, England

# PUBLIC HEALTH AND PRIVATE RIGHTS: HEALTH, SOCIAL AND ETHICAL PERSPECTIVES

Ronald Bayer, Ph.D[1].
Harvey Fineberg, M.D., PhD.[2],
and Thomas Vernon, M.D.[3]

## INTRODUCTION

### Dr. Bayer

Before I turn the podium over to my estimable colleagues, Dr. Fineberg and Dr. Vernon, I'd like to set the tone for this morning's presentations.

The central epidemiological and clinical feature of AIDS, and the feature that makes the public health response to its spread so troubling, is that the transmission of: HTLV-III, LAV, HIV, you have your choice, occurs in the context of the most intimate social relationships, or in contexts that have, for nearly three quarters of a century in the United States proven utterly refractory to social control. The transmission of AIDS occurs in the course of sexual relationship, and in the course of intravenous drug use. In both realms, the evolution of our constitutional law tradition, as well as our social ethos over the past two decades has increasingly recognized the importance of privacy and of limiting state authority. At times we have adopted the position of the importance of privacy on grounds of political philosophy. At times we have done so because of the importance of practicality. It is no accident that the United States Supreme Court discovered what it called the "penumbral" rights of privacy, when dealing with matters of sexuality, and that legal theorists elaborated the notion of a crisis of overcriminalization in discussing public policy and drug use.

It is clear that the only effective public health strategy for the halt of the spread of HTLV-III infection is one that will produce dramatic, perhaps unprecedented changes in the behavior of millions of men and women in this country. Changes in behavior linked to deep biological and psychological drives and desires; changes in behavior that will require acts of restraint and

---

[1] Associate for Policy Studies, The Hastings Center  [2] Dean, Harvard School of Public Health  [3] Executive Director, Colorado Department of Health

deprivation for extended periods, if not for the lives of those infected or at risk for becoming infected. Can we effect such changes? And can we do so in ways that are compatible with our constitutional values?

Faced with the presence of a new infectious and deadly disease, one whose etiologic agent has already infected between one and two million Americans, there is an understandable tendency to believe that the public response ought to bear the marks of the gravity of the situation. A deadly disease, it is held, requires a forceful and even draconian response. The apparent failure, on the part of public health officials, to adopt such a stance has provoked charges of timidity, the subversion of the ethos of public health by that of civil liberties, and even a capitulation to the power of the gay constituency. Such responses may account for: the popularity of certain extremist solutions, the volatility of public opinion polls regarding matters like quarantine and isolation, and the popularity of certain insurgent right wing political groups throughout the country. Of course, fueling these reactions are deeply rooted hostilities towards homosexuality and intravenous drug use. One needn't dismiss the centrality and importance of anxiety around an infectious illness to appreciate how fear of contamination by sexual and behavioral foreigners may amplify social distress.

In this context, some have proposed the mandatory screening of all members of risk groups. Others, the universal screening and surveillance of the entire population. Still others have called for preventive detention with a medical patina: the quarantine of all antibody positive individuals. Clearly all such proposals would tear at the fabric of American social, political, moral and constitutional life. As important, all such proposals, what I call the "Rambo response," would be utterly impractical. How would one screen the entire population, identify all members at risk? How would one adopt a system of surveillance over one to two million individuals? How would one isolate or quarantine such numbers? And how would one retain in confinement those deemed potentially at risk or a threat? More focused are proposals to isolate and quarantine those who behave publicly in ways that put others at risk; the easiest examples being male and female prostitutes who are infected. There are no moral or legal impediments to the restraint of such individuals, but it would be a dangerous illusion to believe that we will break the back of transmission of HTLV-III infection by controlling those who behave publicly in ways that spread this virus. The plain truth is that this virus is spread in the context and in settings that are utterly private, among individuals engaged in consensual sexual activities.

Confronted with the limits, the constitutional and moral limits, as well as the practical limits, of coercive responses, many have turned to education as the solution in the face of HTLV-III transmission. A turn to education, of course, is compatible with our deepest values of civil liberties, privacy, and volunteerism. Unfortunately, the turn to education occurs after more than two decades of experience with the limits of health promotion campaigns. Can anyone look at the data on smoking, alcohol consumption, the use of helmets on the highways by motorcycle drivers, or of seat belts, and believe that health promotion campaigns alone will present a solution to our problems? We have, for close to a year, been given evidence or data of a dramatic change in the behavior of gay men with regard to their sexual activities, and that data has suggested to many that, in fact, in this instance, at any rate, education is working. About three weeks ago, Clad Stevens, of the New York Blood Center, published a study in the Journal of the American Medical Association which is sobering. She did in fact find a dramatic change in the sexual activity of her gay male cohort. The number engaging in anal receptive intercourse dropped from 72 percent to 46 percent. That is a dramatic change in the history of sexual behavior, but it's not good enough. There are some occasions when even dramatic changes lead to disaster.

Where does this leave us? Faced with a fatal illness that has the potential for grave social disruption, the appeals to coercive state police power are seductive, but I believe if pursued, would be socially catastrophic. Confronted with the unacceptable specter of coercion and gross violation of privacy and civil liberties, some have turned to education. Here the risk is that the politically attractive will be confused with the socially efficacious. Between the illusions of power and the illusions of voluntarism it will be necessary to take modest steps that may, by simply slowing the spread of HTLV-III infection, demonstrate, in the language of Albert Camus, "...our commitment to the victims and our commitment to limiting the pestilence..." But at each juncture we must be aware of the fundamental limits of our capacities to fight an infectious disease like AIDS. We are hostage to the advances of virology and immunology, and may be so for many years. The toll will mount in terms of morbidity and mortality, and so will social pressures. The question before us is whether we will be able to meet those pressures with reason and compassion.


DISCUSSION

## Dr. Fineberg

Thank you very much, Ron, and good morning. The subject of this conference, AIDS, is in many ways the paradigmatic public health problem of our time. No disease in modern times has appeared so dramatically, nor called so fully on the resources of our public health institutions, our medical care system and our social institutions. Knowledge about AIDS has been gained from a spectrum of research in the laboratory, in the clinic, and in the field with epidemiological tools. AIDS is a global health problem whose repercussions are being felt and will be felt in countries around the world. The 23 nations represented at this conference testify to the international character of the problem.

In many ways the rapid and wide dissemination of AIDS has depended upon modern technology and upon contemporary lifestyles. It's a disease, after all, that is carried in the person, in one's blood. There is no need for a special climate or a vector or other environmental condition to convey the disease from one place to another. Rapid air transport has facilitated the mixing of populations from one part of the world with those in another. Modern technology to prepare blood products including Factor VIII used in the treatment of hemophiliacs, has permitted international shipment of the disease virus without the host going along. The "sexual revolution" and "gay liberation" are catch words for changes in American lifestyle of the past generation that have greatly enhanced the spread of the AIDS virus.

A central problem in public policy about AIDS is reconciling two frequently conflicting responsibilities of government and the public health community. On the one side, protecting the rights of individuals and on the other side, preserving the health of the public. These dual responsibilities create a fundamental tension that is the principal subject of our session this morning.

Among the rights of individuals which may be threatened by AIDS are the rights to privacy and confidentiality, the freedom to associate with whomever one pleases and the right to nondiscrimination in employment, housing and social services. Individuals whose rights may be threatened as a consequence of AIDS include, of course, patients with AIDS and those with AIDS related complex, also individuals whose blood tests may be positive for antibody to the AIDS virus, and indeed people who are members of high risk groups. The public interests that may be affected by AIDS are of two types. One is a kind of collective economic interest that derives from the costs of care for patients with AIDS. The other is a kind of public interest where the health of members of the public may be threatened, for example by transmission of AIDS from one patient to others in the community.

As policy makers and as health professionals we must be prepared to think simultaneously about the responsibilities to the individual and about responsibilities to the public. In general, all personal privacy rights should not prevail over all public and community rights, nor vice versa. The task of forming intelligent policy is to try in each instance to discern the proper balance when the public and individual interests are in conflict.

In the remainder of my remarks I want to talk about five realities and expectations that condition our approach to the AIDS problem, five principles that I would set forward as guides to policy, and then five recommendations. First, the five realities that should condition our thinking and strategy about dealing with AIDS during the next decade:

Reality No. 1: A reasonable and conservative estimate of the number of patients who will contract clinical AIDS in the next decade is 250,000. Perhaps several million additional patients will require clinical care for less severe symptoms related to infection with the AIDS virus.

Reality No. 2: In the next 10 years the odds are heavily stacked against our having available an effective vaccine or a curative therapy for AIDS. In the case of hepatitis, for example, seven years passed from the concept of the vaccine to the development of a workable vaccine. And 13 years separated the concept from the marketing of a hepatitis vaccine. Even if an AIDS vaccine were created tomorrow, testing for safety and effectiveness would be complicated and consume at least several years, and there is no certainty that a safe and effective vaccine can ever be developed. Successful drug therapy requires both killing all virus, which we know invades the brain, an area protected from many drugs, and reconstituting the patient's immune system. These are formidable requirements unlikely soon to be met. Planning to curtail the epidemic in the next decade should therefore proceed on the assumption that during that time there will be no available vaccine, or effective treatment.

Reality No. 3:  While obviously we must be very concerned with patients who develop clinical AIDS, the greatest challenge to public health is the much larger number of people who carry the virus, yet remain asymptomatic.  We all know the estimates of one to two million Americans who may already have been infected with the AIDS virus.  Most of these people feel healthy and do not know they are infected, neither do their doctors and neither do their sexual partners.  The greatest threat to the health of others emanates from this asymptomatic infected group.

Reality No. 4:  Almost surely, AIDS will continue to spread slowly in the United States heterosexual population.  We've heard already the address from Dr. Clumeck outlining evidence pro and con.  When I use the qualifier "almost surely", I refer both to the fact of spread in the heterosexual population, and to the expected slowness of that spread.  AIDS will come increasingly to be perceived as a disease which is not restricted to high risk populations.

Reality No. 5:  As the number of patients grows and the mix of patients changes, demands for new services and for effective public policies will be felt ever more acutely.  At a national level, policy makers must be sensitive to the marked differences in the distribution of disease and special circumstances in different parts of the United States.  Of course, the value systems and circumstances in different countries will be even more divergent.  The rising wave of cases among intravenous drug users demands special attention, as this will place extreme strain on the network of local and voluntary efforts that have been so effective in supporting patients mainly from the gay population who have contracted the disease.

Now as to principles to guide policy making about AIDS:

Principle No. 1:  Policy decisions about AIDS should be grounded in the best available evidence from science, technology and epidemiology related to the disease.  To illustrate, consider how evidence from such areas as the modes of transmission of the disease and on the performance of diagnostic tests have implications for policy making about the disease.  All available evidence points to the transmission of the AIDS virus among adults through intimate sexual contact or contact with contaminated blood.  The AIDS virus is much less readily transmitted by blood than is the hepatitis virus.  Since the AIDS virus is not transmitted by casual contact, or by air droplets, for example, the rights of children to attend school or of employees to continue working should not be infringed because of unfounded fears on the part of some in the public.

Virtually no diagnostic test is perfect.  Current tests to detect antibody to the AIDS virus are very good, but we can be sure that there will be some errors.  For example, there is a necessary window of time between the exposure to the virus and development of antibodies, during which time an infected patient's blood tested for antibody would be falsely negative.  Related viruses or disease problems could produce false positive results on some tests.  More important, even a very good test loses a great deal of its diagnostic power when it is applied to a population that has a low frequency of infection.  Let me illustrate:  Based on studies of the U.S. blood donor population we may conservatively estimate the frequency of AIDS virus infection in the non-high risk population to be approximately four per 10 thousand. If the ELISA test correctly detects disease 99 percent of the time and correctly rules out disease 99.5 percent of the time, applying a single test to the general population would still produce more than 12 false positive results for every true positive result. Imagine repercussions of screening all couples prior to marriage and informing them of such results. A confirmatory Western blot test that is 99.9 percent specific, and assuming it is fully independent - that is not likely to err in the same way as the initial screening test - would sharply reverse the ratio of true positives to false positives to approximately 70 to one. Yet one or two per hundred falsely confirmed patients is a high price to pay when testing in the general population.

Principle No. 2: Policy makers should contemplate steps that infringe on individual rights only when a path of action can be logically and practically pursued. If, for example, we are contemplating establishing a registry of patients with positive test results, we should ask ourselves what would be done about such patients? Could we follow them in an effective manner? Would the consequences of such a registry, for example, in discouraging people from seeking a test in the first place, be more adverse than positive? These kinds of questions should be answered before advocating steps in public policy that run the risk of infringing upon the rights of individuals.

Principle No. 3: Use the least restrictive means available to protect the community from the threat of the disease. We should try, for example, to have a graded series of responses available to legal authorities to prevent individuals who are potentially infectious from knowingly spreading disease to others. This would apply, for example, to the prostitute and drug addict populations.

Principle No. 4: Government and public health officials must bear in mind the possibility of errors both of commission and of omission in trying to deal with a problem as complicated as AIDS. We should try to learn from our past experiences in efforts to control other infectious diseases, while recognizing that there is no perfect single model from the past and that adjustments to this particular disease and its peculiar features will be necessary.

Principle No. 5: In situations where the collective economic well-being of the public comes into potential conflict with individual rights, such as the case with health insurance, I believe the burden of proof should rest on those who wish to defend the collective public economic welfare. In situations where individuals in the community are placed at risk because of behavior of other individuals, I believe the burden of proof should rest on those who would defend the rights of the individual who by virtue of their actions may inflict harm on others.

Now, let me turn to five policy recommendations:

Recommendation No. 1: The health care system needs to prepare aggressively to care for large numbers of patients with AIDS. This follows simply from the first reality. A special challenge relates to providing adequate social support for patients in such socially disenfranchised categories as drug addicts. Health care for patients with AIDS can be both more compassionate and more efficient through greater reliance on appropriate out-of-hospital and home-care approaches.

Recommendation No.2:  In discharging public responsibility to curtail the epidemic, primary emphasis should be placed on communication and education of an unprecedented magnitude, trying to reach both the public and high risk groups.  By traditional standards of health education, there has been a good deal of effort and a good measure of success informing physicians, patients, some high risk groups and the public at large about AIDS.  Many public and private organizations can justifiably take pride in what they have accomplished.  Yet, when we look at the magnitude of the task before us we have really made only a very small beginning.

We need to think about educating the public in health matters and particularly about AIDS in a wholly new way.  We have to think about it more like a customer oriented corporation views commercial marketing of a new product.  Recently, for example, the Polaroid Corporation introduced a new camera, its Spectra System, and the company reportedly will invest 30 million dollars to make this one product known to the American public.  When Proctor and Gamble introduced New Liquid Tide, a product that was launched with the aid of a household name, the company conducted a new 50 to 60 million dollar promotional campaign.  I am told that when a cigarette company introduces a new brand it expects to spend more than one hundred million dollars around the world to make that brand of "slow death" known to the public.  How much should we be prepared to spend to make health available to the public?  The AIDS epidemic in modern times is an unprecedented threat that warrants a major campaign of accurate, creatively designed communication to reach both the public and high risk groups.

All members of the public need to know enough about AIDS to make informed decisions about their behavior.  We must constantly bear in mind, as Dr. Bayer reminded us, that education to curtail AIDS deals with basic human drives and with the most private of our actions. It is especially important to mount intensive educational efforts in public schools.  Every youth old enough to engage in sexual relations, or to experiment with intravenous drugs needs already to have been educated about AIDS.  Reaching high risk groups in an effective manner will demand determination as well as ingenuity.  IV drug abusers, for example, are the most neglected high risk group still, and pose the greatest threat of transmitting the AIDS virus to the public at large.  I was encouraged to hear Commissioner Axelrod refer to new outreach efforts to get the addict population. Reaching addicts will require an aggressive campaign that goes beyond pamphlets and posters to include face-to-face meetings, straight talk and clear answers.  Speaking of straight talk and clear answers, we in the public health field have to make sure we do not hamstring ourselves more than we already are.  The Centers for Disease Control in its most recent directive about the preparation of materials for group education sessions contains the following guideline and I quote, "Such terms or descriptors used should be those which a reasonable person would conclude should be understood by a broad cross-section of educated adults in society, or which when used to communicate with a specific group like gay men about high risk sexual practices would be judged by a reasonable person to be unoffensive to most educated adults beyond that group".  This kind of restriction on graphic, direct communication is an added handicap that public health officials do not need and that our society can no longer afford.

The public education campaign about AIDS should be based on a comprehensive communication strategy including extensive use of electronic media. At the present time the only federal agency permitted to purchase time on television is the Department of Defense to recruit new soldiers. The United States Congress could improve education on AIDS by providing adequate funds, a minimum of 75 million dollars in the next year and by authorizing the purchase of radio and television time.

Recommendation No. 3: The Public Health Service, I believe, should continue to emphasize voluntary testing of those at risk, and require that counseling be made available to those who test positive and to those who have intimate contact with people who are positive on antibody testing. At this time the preponderance of evidence and logic, I believe, goes against those who would mandate testing in people simply because they are members of a high risk group or who would advocate registration of all who test positive. The safety of our nation's blood supply depends in part on the use of antibody testing. Even more important though, is excluding from blood donation those who are at high risk of carrying the AIDS virus. Alternative anonymous test sites encourage high risk patients to learn their antibody status and to refrain from donating blood simply for that purpose. An additional argument against mandatory testing is the potential for false positive results, as I discussed earlier. The lack of any current, effective therapy, the large numbers of cases, and limited public health resources further argue against routine attempts to trace all contacts of those who test positive. On top of all this is a practical difficulty of establishing and enforcing mandatory testing or follow-up. For example, what would be the frequency of testing? And how would those who test positive be compelled to identify all their contacts? A voluntary system of testing, I believe, bolstered by a new, strong educational effort and counseling service is currently the preferred strategy for limiting the spread of disease.

Recommendation No. 4: My fourth recommendation has already been addressed in part by Dr. Sencer. Methadone maintenance and detoxification facilities must be rapidly expanded to reduce exposure of drug addicts to the lethal AIDS virus. At the present time about 25,000 intravenous drug users are being treated in detoxification and methadone programs in New York City. These programs have long waiting lists, and their numbers could be rapidly expanded by increasing resources devoted to those programs and by making them available at more locations.

Recommendation No. 5: My fifth recommendation relates to the controversy over testing as a criterion for eligibility for health insurance. It is possible, of course, simply to outlaw use of testing as a condition for obtaining health insurance as has been done in a number of states. This approach poses an uncertain risk to insurers who write health insurance and makes them less willing to write insurance in selected geographic areas and for some socioeconomic groups who are deemed to be at high risk. Insurers also argue that this kind of a restriction is contrary to the way in which they currently seek information from patients and examine them for other kinds of health risks, such as hypertension and diabetes. As the number of patients with AIDS continues to grow, the concentration of these patients in certain locales or groups may make it increasingly difficult or impossible for other individuals in those areas or groups to obtain needed health insurance.

Mandatory testing, I believe, is rightly resisted. Testing results would stigmatize people. AIDS is not simply another disease and being labeled as an AIDS carrier, perhaps falsely, is not the same as being a hypertensive.

One solution, I believe, lies in dissolving this controversy by establishing, at the Federal or individual state levels, pools of funds to pay for the cost of medical care of all patients who meet the CDC criteria for AIDS. At a Federal level, this could be accomplished through the Medicare Program (and the need would be eliminated by a national catastrophic insurance plan). At the state level, a funding pool could be underwritten by all licensed insurers who provide health insurance in the state (including government) each paying in proportion to the size of its insured pool.

Establishment of this kind of funding pool would obviate a perceived need for testing of patients among the health insurance industry and would also provide necessary coverage to patients who require it. This proposal would have its own complications, particularly in implementation and in deciding when a patient qualifies as being eligible. The proposal has the advantage of simultaneously providing needed insurance coverage for patients with AIDS, appropriately spreading the cost of care for those patients over all of society, and eliminating the need to rely upon our current, imperfect diagnostic test.

In conclusion, I would say that a comprehensive strategy to deal with AIDS must have many components and approaching the problem will frequently bring individual rights in conflict with the public interest. The aims of this conference, I think, will be well served if through our discussions we can sharpen the development of policies that will deal effectively with the AIDS problem and keep the public and private interests properly in balance. Thank you very much.


### Dr. Vernon

When I began working on my comments for this morning I thought of what an audience might be who would be gathered here. I knew that I represent to some of you the implementer of a controversial public policy in Colorado, and some of you I thought might be suspicious of what Colorado has attempted to do. Others of you may even hope that your states would follow the model that we've adopted. Whatever your perceptions and your experiences as you carry out your own responsibilities in AIDS control, I want to tell you about our experience in Colorado, because here are efforts that we believe are occurring in the traditional model of public health practice to deal with AIDS. Just a note about that environment. We have, very unlike the situation in the city in which we are meeting today, 200 reported cases of AIDS in Colorado since the first case in 1982. To further characterize the environment, I would note that the recently adjourned state legislature granted a grand total of only $100,000 for the control of AIDS in Colorado, money to be dedicated to laboratory services. Unfortunately we did not gain any money for epidemiologic and field work. So we have a very conservative environment relative to the legislature.

I can't tell you that because of what we're doing, we're more wise or going to be more successful than others, but I would like to tell you how we chose the course of action which we have chosen. It's our belief that the qualities and values that are embodied in the traditional model of public health disease control do address the expectations of a fearful public both in hastening the control of this epidemic and in protecting every individual's private rights. We do not believe that this is all of the answer. I accept the contention that has been made by several speakers this morning that we have a problem before us which is different from challenges which we have faced in the past. But it is useful to look at the many victories which have been achieved by public health disease control, perhaps the greatest of which was the eradication of smallpox in recent years.

It's a tragic irony that the same year the smallpox eradication victory was achieved may have been the year that the Human Immunodeficiency Virus (HIV) first came to the United States. It may have been slightly earlier, but the mere coincidence of those two events has been a cause for reflection. Smallpox has been clearly one of the formidible challenges in public health for a very long time and its eradication was accomplished by public health workers and administrators and epidemiologists who understood its mechanisms of transmission and worked with the communities in which that virus spread.

I wouldn't belabor the differences between the two viruses and the two diseases but I do want to note one difference which affects us most profoundly, a difference which is neither virological nor epidemiological: it's that we in public health and in all of society must grapple with ethical, cultural and social beliefs while we do battle with HIV. And, in fact, we have two battles going at the same time. A particularly apt quote from Silverman and Silverman: "At no time in history has a public health crisis and our response to it been so interwoven with human values and attitudes. Never have the social ramifications of our actions been so problematic".

I would note that for one thing we in the western world have not experienced the deep public fear of a seemingly uncontrollable epidemic for over 30 years. One could point to the paralytic polio epidemic prior to Salk and to Sabin. For another, HIV is occurring, as we have noted so many times, in a society where the groups most affected are subject to blame and repression. To quote our moderator and his co-author Carol Levine, I would ask whether we in public health are prepared to grapple with the "one central moral issue. Will the boundaries between private choice and public health responsibility reflect society's concern for the interest of individuals as well as for the common good?"

In addressing this question I found it instructive to examine a set of values that we who practice public health disease control share, whatever our other individual differences may be. First, needless to say, there's a consensus opinion that we are facing the awesome challenge of a lifetime. It may be that the only precedent in our century, to compare with what we are addressing today, was the influenza pandemic of 1918-19, when we lost at least 550,000 people, in only 10 months.

Another value we share is that the proper target for the control of any epidemic, whether it be childhood measles or syphilis, is the agent of that epidemic and the factors which aid the transmission of the agent. It is not general classes or groups of people whose lifestyles are controversial. It is the epidemiologic method which is used to target that agent and I would note that leaders in public health today are not recommending widespread mandatory testing. A third value among us, as public health practitioners, is that a great part of the success of communicable disease control is accomplished by the individuals and communities who are at greatest risk. For example, the near eradication of measles in the United States today is a product of parents deciding to obtain immunizations for their children. The program surely is advanced by the exercise of public health authority through epidemiologic investigations, school immunization laws and immunization record keeping, all of which are critical. But they are effective only with widespread, voluntary, and educated community action. Without prospects for a cure or a vaccine, as Dr. Fineberg noted, we're greatly dependent upon the education efforts of the groups with whom we work. And to date, all across this country much has been accomplished by such groups.

Now, a fourth value, that I addressed earlier, is one that I believe is shared nearly universally. It is that society has a right to protect itself from willful, irresponsible and sociopathic transmission of disease. The majority do have a right to protection from indiscriminate harm from individuals. This protection has been framed in public health statute usually as authority to examine, to isolate or to quarantine. In Colorado as elsewhere the public health statutes relating to this are old and I believe frighteningly broad. They were written in the manner of an earlier society for whom the communicable diseases were a dominant fear. Today, of course, we have adjusted our use of this authority in public health practice. For example, the limited effectiveness of isolation is recognized. Public health practitioners also believe in the necessity for due process and use of the least restrictive means of isolation when all else has failed. But such authority must be utilized to deal with the incorrigible few. I would note that we are talking today in Colorado not simply about the homosexual or female prostitute, but about the individual who is selling plasma from center to center giving a different name each time.

A fifth value that we share is the one I consider of the utmost importance. That is that we must make certain that we protect the rights to privacy and confidentiality. At the heart of our ability to control disease lies a responsibility to protect privacy. It is not only the right thing to do, but it is the practical course of action as well. I do not believe any value is more deeply shared by public health practitioners.

So these are fundamental values that exist among public health practitioners and I believe they have enhanced, and not limited, our successes with measles, with smallpox, with tuberculosis and other communicable diseases. The premise I advance is that public policy and the control of the HIV epidemic are well served by this group of values. A corollary premise is that the public health disease control model deserves the confidence which has been placed in it by the general populace. The expectations placed upon public health in controlling the HIV epidemic are at least as great as in any previous chapter in our history.

Two recent events in Colorado illustrate the application of such values, I believe, to control this epidemic. They received much national attention, much of it critical. But that has seemed to me a small price to pay in comparison with what we believe could happen if public health were to side step its obligation. The first event was the addition to a standing regulation in Colorado requiring the reporting of laboratory HIV antibody tests to the confidential disease control records of the Colorado Department of Health. This was initiated by us last fall shortly after the ELISA and the Western blot tests for HIV antibody were associated with a positive culture for the virus in a high proportion of those concurrently tested. This revelation presented an unexpected disease control opportunity, because it gave us the opportunity to identify and work with the persons most likely to transmit the virus. Colorado's communicable disease control program has long included the confidential reporting by clinical laboratories of some 45 positive findings for about 30 different communicable disease organisms including serologic tests for syphilis which I mention specifically because those tests could also be a marker for sexual preference for those who would attempt to use public records for that purpose. No such attempt has ever been made in Colorado. These reports are submitted to the confidential medical records of the department and are protected by statute, by regulation, by public health intent and by tradition. No identifying information has ever been released from these records, either intentionally or accidentally, to family members, to law enforcement officials, insurers, to employers or any others who on occasion might make inquiries. We're very proud of that record. Of course, once again, as we approached HIV antibody testing and a regulation, we examined our ability to maintain that same total confidentiality, recognizing that we would face pressures which are different from those we have experienced before.

We also had another question which has been asked earlier. Were we risking too much with the regulation that might keep people from being tested? Would any downturn in the testing be a short-term experience? At the time we didn't know. We hoped there wouldn't be any drop, but all we had to go on was a long history of cooperation between public health and high risk groups in Colorado as well as the value of a very good test which provides excellent information to those who are tested.

A third question was whether we would require personal identification of those tested? No. We had no debate on this. The option of not using one's own name has always been available in our disease control programs and HIV testing is no different. Fourth, we asked ourselves whether ethical or legal issues are raised that are different from the reporting of AIDS disease, or different from reporting of other disease agents with identifiers. The ethic appears consistent to us. Very few argue with the reporting of AIDS or of serologic tests for syphilis and the legal precedents are quite clear.

A final consideration, and a very important one, was whether the regulation would benefit disease control. Our answer in Colorado is a firm yes. At its most basic, epidemiology is the orientation of data to time, place and person. Our ability to know the population distribution of characteristics leads to hypotheses concerning etiologic factors. It helps to determine if hypotheses developed in the laboratory or the clinic are consistent with the population distribution of the agent. Without reporting we have less basis for assessing the effectiveness of control measures when they are finally instituted, or more effective ones than we have at the present time. Reporting also provides benefits to individual patients, that we required of any proposed regulation. Skilled counseling is assured. Most individuals who are tested will return to testing sites for competent counseling. Others, at least in the gay community, will receive skilled counseling from friends and colleagues. But there are some who will not, and some who will not return for test results at all, much less receive skillful counseling. With reporting, these individuals too will benefit from confidential follow-up. This is difficult to accomplish in a setting of anonymous testing. There is a third group of people who can benefit from reporting. Those who are contacts of infected persons, but have little or no reason to believe that they have been exposed to the virus. It is clear from many years of experience, in sexually transmitted disease investigations, that skilled interviewers can elicit information that can interrupt a chain of transmission. An uncommon, but often mentioned circumstance would be the child bearing aged woman partner of an infected person for whom the prevention of an in-utero infection is possible. We recognize, even though we are a relatively low incidence state and area, that labor intensive tracing of contacts can be carried out only in a minority of cases, but in that minority of cases we believe that confidential contact tracing will be important in the prevention of disease transmission. I do disagree strongly with Mayor Koch in his contention that it would not be useful.

With these answers the State Board of Health unanimously adopted the addition of the repeatedly positive ELISA test and the positive Western blot test to our laboratory reporting regulations and the decision was widely publicized. The results have been interesting. As the publicity both pro and con peaked, so did voluntary testing. That was in early October and November. But then as we moved into the Thanksgiving and Christmas holiday period, testing dropped off. We suspected it would, and that drop-off may have had something to do - we believe it did drop off - in part because of reportability, but today testing has returned to a steady level of over 100 individuals per week being tested in our facilities in Colorado and to this date we have tested over 6,000 persons. This appears to be more than most states with comparable or larger populations. Some individuals, but apparently not a large number, are using an assumed name when they use the test. Also, I may note to date there have been no pressures from any parties to release any information from our confidential records. We have had no difficulty from inquiries from law enforcement officials or otherwise.

There has been a second Colorado event which I would like to note briefly. It was the introduction of a bill in this winter's general assembly that singles out AIDS control by public health authority. The bill received two labels, both of them unfortunate. The first was the "AIDS Quarantine Bill". After the bill was amended, it became known as the "Gay Rights Bill". Such labels I think are a sign of the polarities between which we work. The bill was not proposed by my department, but rather by a very conservative legislator, known by his colleagues as a member of the John Birch Society. Many predicted that the bill would pass. Our task then was to consult with the legislature in such a way that we could improve upon existing statutes. In the bill we saw an opportunity to strengthen our confidentiality requirements and we requested and achieved an amendment, "Such information shall not be released or made public upon subpoena, search warrant, discovery proceedings or otherwise." We found another opportunity concerning isolation and quarantine. I mentioned earlier that existing Colorado laws were written early in this century and are no longer consistent with the evolution of due process rights and practices. The generic Colorado statute allows us to "...exercise such physical control over property and the persons of the people within this state, as the department may find necessary for the protection of the public health..." I believe this needed to be improved. Thanks to the work of a politically diverse group of legislators including those responsive to gay constituencies the bill was amended in the State Senate to provide criteria for medical isolation, a staged, due process that requires verbal and written warnings prior to any isolation order, a petition recourse, and a court review of each stage. The health department would carry the burden of proof to show probable cause that the orders issued were necessary to protect the public health and that the least restrictive means necessary had been utilized. Well, the bill's outcome was unexpected and I must say ironic. It passed the Senate as amended by a 33 to zero vote. The conservative house sponsor, finding that he could not remove Senate amendments in conference committee, asked his House colleagues to kill the bill. Such a request by a member to kill his own bill is often passed by a unanimous vote. He won by 36 to 29.

So I've described two experiences in Colorado, not to defend them and not to insist, by any means, that the specifics are applicable to all other areas of the country. Indeed, another value we all share is that successful disease control is often specific to the needs and requirements of a local area. I describe these events instead to illustrate how these efforts are occurring within a mainstream of traditional, enlightened public health disease control. It is a mainstream in which are vested the desires and expectations of the society, and they're based upon a history of success of which the eradication of smallpox is a spectacular example. I believe that any failure by public health to attempt to rise to these expectations has special ramifications in the face of the HIV epidemic, because never before have we experienced an epidemic with such an explosive mixture of fear and prejudice. I contend that our best antidote is enlightened, reasoned leadership within a traditional model of public health disease control supplementing all else that we must do. While we continue to examine what right we have to require reporting, to isolate on occasion when necessary, to conduct contact interviews, we must also ask ourselves another question. The public, including many who are at highest risk, have invested us with their trust in the face of a very frightening event. With such an important responsibility do we have the right not to rise to that expectation?


COMMENTS


James Childress, Ph.D. (Kyle Professor of Religious Studies and Professor of Medical Education, University of Virginia)

My field is ethics and I will talk about AIDS from that standpoint. I will assume that the goal of controlling AIDS is a self-evident, moral imperative for societies and individuals alike. Some commentators, not so much here but elsewhere, seem to suggest that this moral imperative cancels or suspends the rest of our moral universe. We often hear the rhetoric, "The AIDS virus has no civil rights". In a strict sense that's true, but the implication of that rhetoric is troubling. That position may not take seriously enough a number of other moral principles and rules that we have to consider in developing public policies to deal with the threat of AIDS. I would like to sketch very quickly elements of an ethical framework that will be similar in many respects to the remarks you have already heard this morning, and then suggest some conditions under which some of these principles and rules can be overridden, and finally offer a few applications.

An ethical framework for thinking about this problem would include the moral imperative of trying to bring AIDS under control. But then there's also a fundamental moral principle of respect for persons. This principle means that we should not treat people merely as means to ends, and from this principle, as well as others, we can derive certain rules that Dr. Fineberg mentioned, including rules of freedom and liberty of action, rules of privacy, and rules of confidentiality. I will not discuss his other rule of nondiscrimination, which is also very important. Now, in most ethical theories these rules are not absolute. They're not mere rules of thumb or maxims or guidelines. They have a lot more weight than that. But they're not absolute. They're rather prima facie binding, or they set presumptions that have to be rebutted even in trying to realize the goal of controlling AIDS. It's necessary for a society to justify overriding or departing from these rules.

Let me sketch four conditions that I think have to be met to justify infringing rules of liberty, privacy or confidentiality. First, it is necessary to show that infringing these rules will probably realize the end of public health that is sought and that the probable benefits of that infringement will outweigh the probable harms, costs, or burdens. This first condition might be called effectiveness and proportionality. A second condition is also, I think, very important. It's not enough to show that infringing these rules will produce better consequences for more people; these rules also direct us to seek alternative ways, short of infringing the rules, to realize the end of public health. If we can protect public health without infringing these moral rules and others, then we should do so. This requirement is one of the last resort or no alternative means, and it would assign priority to educational efforts and other efforts that do not infringe these rules. A third condition, in this ethical framework, would be that even when society justifiably infringes these rules in order to protect the public health, it should seek policies that least infringe these rules. That is, only the infringement that is necessary to realize the end is acceptable. Let's call this third condition that of least infringement. Now, it would work out in slightly different language for the different moral rules. When we're talking about liberty of action, we should seek the least restrictive alternative. when we're talking about privacy, we should seek the least intrusive option. When we're talking about confidentiality, we should seek the course of action that would involve the least disclosure of information. Those are three conditions that I think are very important. A fourth condition would apply even when we justifiably infringe the moral rules in question. That is, when we think that the conditions of effectiveness and proportionality, last resort, and least infringement have all been met, we still are required by the principle of respect for persons to inform the person whose liberty, or privacy, or confidential relations have been infringed. Sissela Bok has noted that in some contexts, secret or deceptive action may be more disrespectful of persons than coercive action. I would suggest that we may be required, by the principle of respect for persons, to disclose the action to the person involved, to justify the action to that person, and perhaps even in some cases to engage in compensatory measures.

With that ethical framework with its principles and rules and conditions for justified infringement of those rules, let me make a few comments about application. For example, if we consider screening for antibodies that indicate exposure to the HTLV-III/LAV virus we can chart possible screening policies in terms of the degree of voluntariness from voluntary to mandatory or compulsory. And we can chart such policies in terms of the extent of screening--whether it's selective or universal. I think the arguments that we've heard today stand against universal mass screening, voluntary or compulsory. I think that mass screening of either form really doesn't satisfy the conditions I sketched. Regarding selective screening, whether voluntary or mandatory, I think we need to draw some distinctions. I think that voluntary screening certainly should be available for those who want it. And they should not, in effect, have incentives to try to donate blood in order to obtain that screening. However, there's a lot more debate than perhaps has been suggested today about whether voluntary screening of people in high risk groups should be encouraged, in part because of questions about what should be done after the screening has been conducted. Basically we have a couple of different models. One model would be to test people and then to counsel those with positive results to change their behavior. And if the recommendations would be the same in either case, it may still be debatable as to what extent voluntary screening of people, even in high risk groups, should be encouraged.

Now regarding compulsory selective screening, I think there are some areas in which we feel quite comfortable with mandatory screening, for example, of people who want to donate blood, or sperm, or organs. If they choose to engage in that act of donation then mandatory screening is appropriate. It's less clear that it is appropriate in a number of other settings, such as employment. Let me comment specifically on insurance since it has already come up today. I agree with the general direction that at least two previous speakers have emphasized. We should think about screening for health insurance less in terms of what insurance companies are obligated to do and more in terms of what the society is obligated to do. We should face the question directly--is there a societal obligation to provide health care in this area, with the federal government providing the primary resources. I would prefer to see us confront this issue directly, rather than concentrating on the obligations of insurance companies.

Once information has been obtained by voluntary screening or mandatory screening in a few selected areas, what should be done with it? What is its value? What is its point? Now, first of all this is a question about disclosure of information to the patient. (I'm using the term "patient" here to refer to one who has been exposed to the virus, who tests antibody positive, and not simply one who has AIDS.) There's general agreement that the patient has a right to know. There's more controversy--we may want to come back to this later today--about whether the patient has a right not to know. But then there is also the problem of disclosure to others. Some of our discussion today has already focused on legally required disclosure of information to public health officials beyond the requirement to report AIDS, for example, the requirement in Colorado to report positive results on the antibody test. We've heard some of the reasons for that policy ably presented by Dr. Vernon. I think there are some questions about whether reporting itself should be mandatory, if screening remains optional, though perhaps encouraged. If screening is optional, people may worry about what will happen with that information and refrain from participation. So it's not clear how effective this policy will be in the overall control of the problem without compulsory universal screening--about which I've already raised questions--or without some means other than education. Then there are questions about breaches of confidentiality to protect other individuals, contact tracing, etc. I think that breaches of confidentiality can be justified in some settings. The larger anxiety about the disclosure of information has to do with unjustified breaches of confidentiality. What will happen to the information apart from the breaches that might be justified? In one case a physician called a positive test result into the patient's office, leaving the result with the secretary because the patient was out, and the patient received the report at the same time he received the notice that he was fired. Such breaches, whether deliberate or careless, must be avoided because they create major social costs for the victims without any compensating benefits.

My final remark concerns the problem of moralism and legalism in our debates about public policies in this area. Moralism and legalism have blocked our search for effective ways to deal with AIDS as a threat to public health. One philosopher described moralism as "deformed morality" and legalism as "deformed legality". How have they stood in the way? We've already heard examples today. Also recall widespread comments about the "gay plague" as well as various efforts to blame victims. Notice the widespread language about guilt and innocence. Moralism and legalism have also stood in the way, for example, of the government promoting "safe sex" because sex among homosexuals is often viewed as illicit, sometimes as illegal and certainly as immoral. We've heard about the requirement that the terms in education be "unoffensive" to people outside of the high risk groups. I think that moralism and legalism have also appeared in the debate about the provision of needles and syringes for intravenous drug users. In short, I think we need to move beyond moralism and legalism in order to pay attention to some of our important moral values of liberty, privacy, confidentiality and respect for persons as we pursue this morally imperative goal of reducing the threat of AIDS. Thank you very much.


Dean Echenberg, M.D., Ph.D. (Director, Bureau of Communicable Disease Control, Department of Public Health, City and County of San Francisco)

We have heard some rather dramatic contrasts in approaches to AIDS prevention here this morning. We heard Mayor Koch talking about contact tracing as something that should be almost flippantly dismissed, and then we heard Dr. Vernon talk about a contact tracing program that has been set up in Colorado. I think it might be helpful to take a look at the history of this epidemic because I think it sheds some light on how both approaches may be right depending on the situation. As usual we're always trying to find some sort of a simplistic or universal approach to control this epidemic. There's not one way to treat any disease. There's not one way to deal with this epidemic.

We can learn a great deal about our modes of intervention and get some perspective by seeing how this epidemic started in San Francisco. We've been following a cohort of homosexual men in San Francisco since 1979. Originally, they volunteered for testing Hepatitis B vaccines. In 1984 we realized that many of these men were infected with the AIDS Virus. We asked them to volunteer for AIDS studies and examined their bloods from 1979.

One of the most tragic statistics in this overall tragedy is that by the time the first article appeared in print in the MMWR in July 1981, 30 to 40 percent of this cohort was already infected. That's how much of a jump this virus had on us before we even knew it was there. It took another six months to a year before we understood the mode of transmission, at which time 40 to 50 percent of the cohort was infected.

The strategies that evolved to deal with this type of situation in San Francisco were obviously very different than the strategies that one uses in a situation today where the prevalence is much lower.

In San Francisco and through most of the country, in the initial stages of the epidemic, a strategy evolved that in effect said that all those people in the classic high risk group should consider themselves infectious through sexual contact. This not only included gay men, but it also included hemophiliacs and IV drug users. This approach which utilizes a strategy of mass education has been relatively effective. Mass education has had a great impact in decreasing the level of unsafe sexual activities that can transmit the virus. We used to see 500 cases of rectal gonorrhea in San Francisco at our sexually transmitted disease clinic each month. It has now decreased to less than 50 per month. The drop started soon after the first MMWR articles were published.

When we began to see cases outside the classic high risk groups different strategies were needed. Fifty percent of the gay men in San Francisco are infected. In the general heterosexual population the prevalence is less than a fraction of one percent. Nevertheless in this latter case, the progress of the epidemic might be even more insidious because these heterosexuals often won't know they are infected. The incubation period for AIDS can be up to seven years and possibly longer. An infected individual might be able to carry this virus and infect others unknowingly all this time. We cannot assume that we're going to see the same kind of decrease in unsafe sexual activity in the heterosexual population. The immediacy of the epidemic among heterosexuals is very different.

I think an attempt to find individuals who are infectious and don't know it is a reasonable way to proceed. That is what we have done in San Francisco. Thus we are dealing with both a high prevalence group, and a very low prevalence group. In the former we are using a mass education campaign and in the latter we have started a contact tracing and a partner referral program.

We have a very high degree of cooperation. The program has been relatively successful. It's completely voluntary. These programs are based on the assumption that no one wants to infect another person unknowingly. We try to find people who are infected and don't know it. We ask anyone who has been diagnosed with AIDS to give us the names of their heterosexual partners so that we can contact them and explain to them what the situation is. Once we explain the program, we use very sensitive investigators who have had long experience dealing with the community in San Francisco. We have a very high degree of cooperation. If an individual says that they would rather tell their partner themselves, that's fine. If, in some cases they'd rather not participate, that's also their prerogative. With this program we have located quite a number of women who were infectious (who were infected) and didn't know it.

I think that there are a couple of reasons why we could do this in San Francisco. State Assemblyman Art Agnos was very instrumental in passing a law that makes it illegal to give information about anybody's antibody status without written consent. Without that law I don't know if we would have been able to have a program like this. I think that it's extremely important for anyone who's contemplating these kinds of programs to understand the essential confidentiality needed. There must be very strong legal protections to safeguard this information from all subpoenas.

To sum up, this is an international conference and I think each country and each locality is going to have to look at their own epidemiology. They must determine what is happening in their own communities and design their own interventions. They can't expect to take the programs that have worked in other places and import them whole. It's going to have to be a local response based on the local situation. In some situations where the prevalence is extremely high, contact tracing is inefficient and inappropriate. On the other hand, where the number of cases is small, where there are safeguards on confidentiality and sensitive case counselors, contact tracing and partner referral can play an important role in dealing with the AIDS epidemic.


Michael Adler, M.D. (Chairman, Department of Genito-Urinary Medicine, Middlesex Hospital Medical School, London, England)

Thank you very much, indeed. I'd like to respond to some of the things I've heard this morning. I'd like to start by making some general comments about the balance between the private individual and public health. And then maybe I could just say a little bit about confidentiality and notification in the United Kingdom, and also respond to Dean's remarks about contact tracing. I was rather concerned this morning, when I was sitting in the audience, that people felt that reason will prevail in terms of the balance between the rights of the private individual and what we have to do to contain this disease as a public health issue. I was concerned that the remarks might lull us all into a false sense of inertia and that we will rest on our mental laurels. Now, I may be wrong, but I think that this tension is very important; the tension between the protection of the public health and the protection of the individual. Where you stand on this spectrum depends a little bit upon your personal interest. It seems to me that, as a patient, or as a potential patient, your primary concern is that you will be treated sympathetically and that all the traditions of the doctor/patient relationship will prevail, i.e. confidentiality and that you will be able to retain your basic human rights until you

die.  Now, as a general member of society one may respond very
differently to this and feel that containment through quarantine and
notification are the most important aspects of control and should
completely override an individual's liberty and freedom of choice.
It seems to me that all of us in this room do not have an opinion
that is markedly different from the opinion and perspective of the
patient.  We're all talking to each other and thinking along the
same lines.  I think that's dangerous.  I think it's dangerous
because I think that logic will not necessarily prevail unless we
discuss the issues among ourselves.  I think that the politicians
will get into the act much more avidly and in a much more
reactionary way than they have to date.  We have begun to see this
in the United Kingdom.  And I fail to believe that you are not
seeing this this here in the United States.  But as each month goes
by and we all are failing to, ar seem to be failing to
control AIDS and HTLV-III infection, the political pressure will
increase.  It will increase even more when this "condition", as
Nathan Clumeck has decribed it this morning, gets into the
heterosexual community, which I believe it will.  Once it is a
heterosexual disease and once one sees perinatal transmission no one
will be able to escape the reality of AIDS.  We will not be able to
use the normal defense mechanisms that we have seen in society -
that of rejecting it.  I am concerned that we, as professionals,
should try and review all the public health and ethical issues that
we feel are inappropriate, such as quarantine.  We've heard that
policy makers should only infringe public rights when logically
pursued.  I think as professionals we have to show that it would be
illogical to do certain things.  We need to rehearse those arguments
now, so that we're prepared for illogical responses that are going
to be politically motivated.  We have seen this in the United
Kingdom in relation to a very simple issue, namely notification of
AIDS.  At present in the United Kingdom AIDS is not a notifiable
disease, and notification is purely voluntary.  But about 18 months
ago politicians were concerned that it should become notifiable.
And the reason why they were concerned was that they wished to be
seen as doing something and as having a grip on the situation.  It
took a very strong argument, hopefully it was a logical argument, to
persuade them that this was not appropriate.  But that argument will
rise again in 18 months or in two years.

Maybe I could finish by saying a few words about contact tracing
in the United Kingdom.  In general terms it's true to say that we
have rejected the concept that one should contact trace in HTLV-III
infection, primarily because there is no treatment available.  It is
unlike any other sexually transmitted disease such as syphilis and
gonorrhea where contact tracing is effective in that you can treat
and you can prevent complications.  Now, we've heard from Dean a
scenario which would suggest that if you contact trace you can break
a chain of transmission.  And here I think we're in a situation
where you're balancing the good of the public health against what is
right and good for the individual.  I don't know what the answer is,
but we all know that there are major disadvantages and disbenefits
to the individual of knowing that they're antibody positive both in
social and psychiatric morbidity.  I think we have to ask ourselves,
is that morbidity assuaged by the new knowledge that you give to the
individual, i.e. that if they alter their behavior they will
actually stop infecting others?  Thank you.

Session B:   Research:   International Cooperation and Competition

<u>Participants</u>

<u>Speakers</u>

James Wyngaarden, M.D.
Director, National Institutes of Health

Julian Gold, M.D.
Director, Sydney AIDS Center, Sydney, Australia

<u>Panelists</u>

LeRoy Walters, Ph.D.
Director, Center for Bioethics, Kennedy Institute of Ethics

Morris Abram, J.D.
Former Chairman of the President's Commission on the Study of
Medical Ethics, Vice Chairman, Civil Rights Commission

Andrew Moss, Ph.D.
Adjunct Assistant Professor, Department of Epidemiology and
International Health, University of California, San Francisco

John Seale. M.D., M.R.C.P.
Venereologist, London, England

Susan Zolla-Pazner, Ph.D.
Co-Director, AIDS Center, Manhattan VA Medical Center

# RESEARCH: INTERNATIONAL COOPERATION AND COMPETITION

LeRoy Walters, Ph.D.[1],
James Wyngaarden, M.D.[2], and
Julian Gold, M.D.[3]

## INTRODUCTION

### Dr. Walters

This panel this afternoon will be devoted to research questions. We've taken a very broad definition of research. It includes at least four elements.

One is basic laboratory research on such matters as how retroviruses function. A second aspect of research is epidemiologic research. A third is pre-clinical studies, that is, targeted research directed toward the development of chemotherapies or vaccines. And a final stage of research is clinical trials of chemotherapies or vaccines.

I hope that you will notice during our discussions this afternoon, and we're also noticing this morning, what kinds of metaphors or analogies are used to illustrate the AIDS problem. For example, I think we heard the following analogies cited during one or another part of the discussion this morning. AIDS is somewhat like genital herpes, syphilis, smallpox, influenza (early in this century), polio, hepatitis B or retroviral infections in certain species of monkeys or in sheep or goats. All of these are analogies in one respect or another. Similarly, you may try to keep in mind what analogies might be appropriate for the response that our society ought to take in dealing with the AIDS question.

Might we need something in the scale of the Manhattan Project, or the Apollo Moon Project, or the war on cancer or the Space Shuttle Program?

---

[1] Director, Center for Bioethics, Kennedy Institute of Ethics
[2] Director, National Institutes of Health [3] Director, Sydney AIDS Center, Sydney, Australia

# DISCUSSION

## Dr. Wyngaarden

I am very happy to have the opportunity to participate in this session on international cooperation in AIDS research. Continued international collaboration is vital if we are to maintain our momentum toward conquering AIDS, particularly because epidemiological studies outside of the U.S. are beginning to provide tantalizing clues that may lead us to a better understanding of transmission of the causative agent and contribute to strategies for preventing the disease - now recognized as a problem worldwide.

As many of you know, NIH's commitment to international cooperation in research goes back to its very origins. As NIH approaches its centennial anniversary, and we begin to delve into our history, it has become clear that many of the basic principles upon which NIH was founded are sustained today. One of these tenets is the recognition that biomedical research knows no geographical or political boundaries. In fact, our predecessor organization - the Laboratory of Hygiene - was established on Staten Island in 1887 because the Congress felt it necessary to create a research laboratory to study diseases that were international in scope and that had serious effects in the United States. Among these were cholera, yellow fever, and tuberculosis. Because European Laboratories were at the time the recognized leaders in biomedical research, the first Director of the Laboratory of Hygiene, Dr. Joseph Kinyoun, traveled to Europe to study under Dr. Robert Koch, where he learned the new techniques for isolation and identification of bacteria, and to the Pasteur Institute in France, where he studied methods of preventing rabies. So from its very beginning, NIH has been cognizant of the international nature of biomedical research and has sought to encourage and foster both formal and informal cooperative research efforts.

Many of NIH's programs to enhance international cooperation in biomedical research are focused in its Fogarty International Center (FIC), established in 1968. Through its International Studies Program, FIC addresses problems concerning international aspects of biomedical and behavioral research, research manpower training, and the transfer of research results. Examples of work conducted under this program include a series of international studies to evaluate available research and its potential applicability to eradicate diseases including measles, polio, and yaws. Other recent collaborative efforts include a meeting on state-of-the-art research related to oncogenes, cell growth, and cancer, and a conference on information processing and medical imaging that brought together 100 researchers from five continents.

The FIC Scholars-in-Residence Program, mandated in 1967, enables distinguished scientists and established scholars to interact with NIH intramural scientists for periods of up to one year on subjects relating to international health. These senior scientists, the majority from western Europe, North America, Japan, and Asia, help to establish points of collaboration between institutions in various countries. It was through this progam that Dr. William Jarrett, a well-known expert on animal retroviruses from Glasgow, came to work with NIH scientists studying the development of antibodies to various components of the AIDS virus. Dr. Ian Gust, Director of the Medical Research Center at the Fairfield Hospital in Melbourne, is another FIC Scholar concentrating on AIDS. His observations about the pattern of AIDS in Australia have been intriguing to NIH scientists because it differs dramatically from the pattern in the U.S. In Australia, a higher fraction of AIDS cases arise from blood transfusion, while there are very few cases as a result of IV drug use.

Other FIC programs bring foreign postdoctoral scientists to the United States to work with U.S. scientists on problems of mutual interest and send U.S. scientists abroad for study. Some 100 foreign scientists are brought here annually under this program, while approximately 50 U.S. researchers are sent abroad each year.

The NIH intramural research program also attracts talented scientists from around the world, who come to Bethesda to share in the resources of the NIH. Distinguished scientists at varying levels in their careers are invited to receive further training or to conduct research in their biomedical specialities. Stipends are provided, and each participant in the visiting program works closely with a senior NIH investigator who serves as sponsor or supervisor during the visitor's period of appointment. Currently, more than 1,100 scientists from 70 countries are participating in our visitors' programs, with highest representation from Japan, the United Kingdom, Italy, India, and Israel. An additional 400 guest workers also participate in research at the NIH, getting laboratory space and research support, but no stipend. These programs, over the years, have created an international network of scientists who continue to collaborate with their NIH counterparts throughout their scientific careers. At present, there are 25 foreign nationals working in collaboration with NIH scientists in the two NIH laboratories that are devoted entirely to AIDS research.

In addition to these programs, which operate primarily through the Fogarty International Center, the individual research institutes of NIH all engage in international projects that take advantage of research opportunities existing abroad. These projects and programs contribute not only to our scientific knowledge base, but also to improving health in the geographic area of interest. Well-known examples include the work of NIH's Dr. Carleton Gajdusek on the slow virus causing the disease kuru in New Guinea. His field studies earned him the Nobel Prize in Medicine or Physiology in 1976 and provided insights into other neurological diseases believed to be caused by slow viruses. Another example is the NIH study at Lake Maracaibo, Venezuela, where an extended family of 3,000 with a very high rate of Huntington's Disease has been identified. This Venezuela family represents the largest living concentration of the genetic disease in the world and is a great resource in the search for the defective gene in Huntington's Disease.

Similar opportunities seem to exist with regard to AIDS, particularly in certain parts of Africa. But before discussing those epidemiological findings, I would like to provide a bit of background on NIH's overall efforts in approaching the AIDS problem.

Despite early criticism to the contrary, NIH was quick to apply its particular expertise and resources to the AIDS problem; our follow up to international aspects of the disease has been equally swift.

The NIH and the scientific community in this country have been able to respond to AIDS in a remarkable way because of an enormous investment in fundamental research over the years. By the time the first AIDS cases were recognized in March and April of 1981 - by scientists at UCLA supported by the NIH - that prior investment in basic research had already generated a wealth of fundamental knowledge in such areas as immunoregulation, basic virology, opportunistic pathogens, the retroviruses, and DNA recombination. Without the benefit of these modern understandings and technologies, it would have been impossible even to identify and characterize AIDS. In addition, a long standing national commitment to training research scientists - both M.D.'s and PhD's assured a cadre of prepared researchers around the country who were ready to apply their expertise to the challenges posed by AIDS.

With these resources in place, along with a strong intramural research program, NIH was prepared to respond quickly to the emerging epidemic.

The NIH intramural research program was prepared to take an early lead, partly because intramural resources are administratively easier to refocus than extramural mechanisms and partly because NIH was fortuitously endowed with recognized experts in areas related to AIDS. Dr. Anthony Fauci, now Director of the National Institute of Allergy and Infectious Diseases, at that time was chief of NIAID's Laboratory of Immunoregulation, as well as an authority on the immune system in health and disease. The other major figure was Dr. Robert Gallo, of The National Cancer Institute (NCI), who in 1979 had reported the first isolation of a human RNA tumor virus, called HTLV-I, which apparently was associated with adult T-cell leukemia and acquired by infection rather than genetic transmission. Dr. Gallo built this major advance upon his earlier work - the discovery of T-cell growth factor (now called interleukin 2) - which enabled the long-term culture of relatively mature T-cells, which in turn enabled the identification of HTLV-I in T-cell lymphoma cell lines. But the significance of Dr. Gallo's findings could not have been explored absent international collaborations. The availability of Gallo's system offered the opportunity for seroepidemiologic studies demonstrating the endemic nature of HTLV-I in areas of Japan, the West Indies, Southeast USA, China, the USSR, Africa, Malaysia, and Central and South America. Although adult T-cell leukemia does not rank as a major health problem in the United States, the contributions Dr. Gallo made to our basic knowledge about retroviruses obviously were enormous. Shortly thereafter, as Dr. Gallo turned his attention toward the problem of AIDS, the payoff was rapid.

Early on, the NIH included the extramural community in accelerated efforts to learn about the new disease. Supplemental awards were made by the NCI to scientists already supported by NIH so that their research could be redirected toward AIDS. This early effort to encourage research on AIDS by extramural investigators required diverting funds from other NIH progams because no money had been appropriated for AIDS research.

A number of workshops were held to bring together NIH researchers and scientists nationwide - with recognized experts from abroad - to discuss preliminary research leads and to develop a course of research action. While the scientific community began to initiate studies on the causes of AIDS and some outstanding researchers turned their attention to the problem, NIH began to stimulate research on various aspects of AIDS through issuance of specific Requests for Applications.

Research advances rapidly followed the discovery of the causative agent for AIDS. They included: a description of the underlying immune defects characteristic of the disease; the development of tests for screening donated blood; improved understanding of the modes of transmission; development of methods for processing blood products used by hemophiliacs; complete deciphering of the genetic code of the causative virus; and recognition that the brain is a primary site of infection. We have also learned a great deal about how the virus infects cells, about the antibodies produced by most people infected with the virus, and about the mechanisms by which the virus propagates. Many of these advances have laid important groundwork for our current challenges: development of therapeutic agents and vaccines.

In terms of budgetary response, funding for AIDS has expanded rapidly. In 1982, the Public Health Service allocated $5.5 million for AIDS programs, with $3.4 million for NIH; in 1986, NIH's total obligation for AIDS research is estimated at about $134 million. It is interesting to note the change in the proportion of funds spent on AIDS intramurally and in extramural programs over the past five years - in 1982, 53 percent of the funds were spent on intramural AIDS studies and 47 percent extramurally. By 1986 the proportions had gradually shifted so that only 23 percent of the now much larger AIDS budget is allocated to intramural studies while 77 percent is allocated to extramural projects. The change in the relative proportions - intramural to extramural - is seen as a natural evolution reflecting increased interest in AIDS research within the scientific community.

At present, NIH's AIDS research program is emphasizing the development of agents to treat the disease and vaccines to prevent it, with adjuvant studies of basic research on pathogenesis and natural history.

The Public Health Service, through both NIH and the Centers for Disease Control (CDC), has been interested in doing epidemiologic studies of AIDS in various parts of Africa since 1983 when clinicians in Brussels and Paris reported AIDS-like illnesses and T-cell abnormalities among African patients without any known lifestyle risk factors for AIDS. These observations led investigators to Rwanda and Zaire, where the patients seen in Belgium had lived and where other patients with similar abnormalities were discovered. After the causative retrovirus for AIDS was determined, studies in Africa quickly confirmed that the same virus was causing the disease in Africa as in the U.S. and Europe.

The data gathered from African population studies thus far are providing clues as to the emergence of AIDS in that continent. These studies are important because if HTLV-III/LAV and AIDS are new to Africa and only now being disseminated, then it becomes urgent from a public health standpoint to understand the mechanisms by which this agent is being spread and to institute control measures.

The NIH is currently supporting, in collaboration with the CDC, a project to study AIDS in Zaire. Studies in African populations have great importance in better understanding the disease in the United States. In contrast to the United States, where most cases are in homosexual males, the ratio of male to female cases in Zaire is 1:1, and there is strong evidence for heterosexual transmission. Information on the transmission of the disease in Africa may be an important indicator of the potential for a greater degree of heterosexual transmission in the U.S. In addition, studies of the cofactors involved in the development of AIDS in Africa may give clues to cofactors involved in the disease elsewhere.

The search in Africa for a progenitor agent from which the AIDS virus may have mutated or with which it may have recombined is also of critical importance. Studies of the differences between this ancestor virus and the current AIDS agent could provide data that would indicate which portion of the genome confers the pathogenic potential, information that would be useful in designing better therapies for AIDS. In addition, the non-pathogenic progenitor could be examined as a source for a safe immunizing material provided there is any neutralizing cross-reactivity between the two agents. To date, this putative progenitor has not been identified, although there is some evidence pointing toward an agent in African green monkey which is cross-reactive with HTLV-III/LAV.

Additional NIH-supported studies are beginning in prostitutes in Kenya, with direct relevance to similar studies being conducted within the U.S. In the next few years, NIH expects to undertake several other important studies in other countries: natural history studies in homosexual populations in the Caribbean and in Asia (Thailand and Singapore); natural history studies of heterosexually transmitted AIDS in Zaire; prospective studies of AIDS in female prostitutes in Kenya, Trinidad, Jamaica, Surinam, Zambia and Thailand; studies of vertical transmission from mother to newborn, which is common in Africa; studies on cofactors such as parasitic infections and their role in the development of the disease; the identification of nonhuman primate reservoirs in Africa; and studies of racial/genetic factors that may influence acquisition of infection and expressions of disease, for example, studies of the unexplained difference in the rate of disease in those of African versus Asian descent in Trinidad.

In conclusion, international cooperation has been a feature of AIDS research dating from the time the syndrome was recognized as an infectious disease, not only because of the obvious public health issue involved, but also because of the nature of biomedical research and a tradition that demands that scientists be constantly up to date on the cumulative knowledge base in their fields.

International conferences have always been fruitful mechanisms for the interchange of ideas in biomedical research, and this has been the case for scientific subjects relating to AIDS. For example, in January of this year, the NIH and the Association pour la Recherche sur le Cancer sponsored an international symposium in Martinique on virus-associated cancers, bringing together many world renowned virologists, epidemiologists and clinicians concerned with retrovirus research. This meeting was an extension of a similar symposium sponsored by the French institution on virus-associated cancers in Africa. A number of international conferences specifically aimed at bringing together scientists concerned with AIDS have been held over the past five years. For example, in 1983, the Pan American Health Organization and the NIAID sponsored a regional meeting on AIDS in the Americas which included public health officials from North, South and Central America. Just last week in Bethesda, NIH epidemiologists participated in a workshop on AIDS in Africa set up by the Armed Forces Institute of Pathology.

Many of you are already aware of the First International Conference on AIDS held in Atlanta in 1985, sponsored primarily by the U.S. Public Health Service with assistance from WHO. The Second International Conference on AIDS, which will draw a large number of U.S. scientists, is to be held next month in Paris, primarily sponsored by French institutions. NIH will be the location for the Third International Conference on AIDS, to be held in June of 1987. Planning for that meeting is already underway.

Another formal mechanism to encourage international cooperation on AIDS is set up by WHO. NIH, the Centers for Disease Control, and the Food and Drug Administration, as well as other organizations around the world are formally recognized as WHO collaborating centers on AIDS, responsible primarily for enhancing information exchange aimed at developing international collaboration, training of laboratory personnel in specialized techniques, providing reference reagents, evaluating diagnostic tests, and organizing activities to determine the natural history of the disease in different parts of the world.


## Dr. Gold

Thank you very much for inviting me here to speak on AIDS research, cooperation and competition. It's been almost five years since I worked here at the New York City Health Department and in retrospect it seems that I left just when the first young man was being diagnosed as having AIDS. Prior to that, during the three and a half years I was based at the Centers for Disease Control in Atlanta, and then here in New York, I had an opportunity to conduct many investigations around the country. It's become clear to me that in many ways Australia and especially Sydney, the largest city, represents a microcosm of U.S. cities like San Francisco, Los Angeles, and to a lesser extent, New York City.

In this talk I would like to draw on the similarities and differences between our two countries, to focus on aspects of research into the natural history of the AIDS virus. I will concentrate on cooperation in epidemiological and behavioral research, rather than on laboratory based immunology or virology, because Australia is not at the forefront of these endeavors and because in our day-to-day clinical work, no matter where we practice, the ultrastructural advances, as brilliant and interesting as they are, have had little if any impact on the prognosis or management of our patients. Over the past 10 years our society has learned bitter lessons about medical research. After the dramas of thalidomide, the intrauterine device and DES, no one could argue that any measures to protect the physical or mental well-being of study subjects are appropriate and indeed essential. However, in our genuine concern to ensure that this

protection is above reproach, especially above litigation based
reproach, we have adopted severe and in some cases
counterproductive research methodologies that may be helping to
spread the AIDS virus rather than stopping it.

I find it interesting that in the privacy of the face-to-face
doctor/patient setting, where our responsibility is to the
individual alone, we are free to ask any questions about lifestyle,
behavior or sexual practices that may be relevant in deciding
treatment not only in relation to AIDS, but in medical and
counseling practice overall.  So long as the information goes no
further than the scribbled notes of the medical record, both the
patient and doctor feel protected.  But once we start to fill in a
data collection instrument and the words "computer analysis" are
mentioned, even though the questions may be exactly the same as
those asked in the clinical setting I just mentioned, both the
patient and doctor feel threatened.  We are worried about
confidentiality and privacy, and question the intentions of people
who want access to any data.  I wonder how much valuable
information is locked away, unuseable, in the medical record vaults
of our major hospitals and clinical practices.  Thus an underlying
theme of this paper is to propose a model service that straddles
the gap between clinical care and research, such that each piece of
information gleaned from the individual is used to help the group.
The group, in this case, are people who have been infected with the
AIDS virus and the model is one that has now been in place for just
over a year at the Sydney AIDS Clinic.  However, before launching
into the specifics of our clinical observations/research, I would
like to put the AIDS situation in Australia into some perspective
for you.

Although Australia and the United States are geographically
about the same size, we have less than seven percent of your
population and more than 90 percent of them are crowded into five
cities around our coast.  Those of you who have been to Australia's
capital cities will appreciate that urban lifestyles and social
structure are very similar to here.  We estimate that by comparing
the population based case rates, the pattern of AIDS in Australia
may be three years behind the United States, thus we all have an
opportunity to test whether the old adage, "If we could have only
done that two or three years ago," really works in relation to the
AIDS epidemic.  In other words, Australia could be seen as an
experimental model, as yet unaffected by the terrible toll that
AIDS has taken on victims and health workers alike.  In this
respect, research collaboration between these two epidemic time
zones should be seen as an important priority.  Homosexual or
bisexual men make up about 86 percent of Australian cases, compared
with 72 percent here.  The first 20 cases in gay men in Sydney had
probably become infected following trips to the west coast of the
United States during the early 1980s.  It wasn't until 1984 that
the first indigenously acquired case was reported.  The number of
cases of AIDS among blood product recipients in Australia is
relatively five times higher than here.  Perhaps the most important
stimulus to government and public attention over the AIDS situation
came in late 1984 when four babies in Queensland were shown to have
died of transfusion associated AIDS all from a single donor.  The
government response nationally was to introduce a legally binding
donor declaration form for high risk groups; pour most of the
allocated AIDS funding into ensuring safety of the blood
transfusion system, and to mount an extensive public information

campaign to convince people that it's really alright to swim in pools, to eat in restaurants and to have a haircut. While these initiatives are very important, they have done little to interrupt the epidemic. For example, for the seven million dollars already spent on donor screening in Australia, 29 positive donors have been found at a cost of $250,000 each. As well, even the public education campaigns have waned in direct proportion to the amount of media coverage on the AIDS issue. Of the 1.5 million dollars allocated to AIDS research in Australia in 1986, almost 80 percent has gone to buy equipment and to conduct highly technical laboratory based research. It has been very difficult for us to convince the highly respected quorums of medical professors that research in relation to AIDS is not necessarily, absolutely synonymous with an electron microscope of a Coulter T-cell counter. While we continue to discuss AIDS, the number of cases continues to rise. There are 22 different government AIDS committees in Australia and they meet about 70 times a year.

As with the United States, the highest number of AIDS cases are concentrated in a few centers. Almost 70 percent are in New South Wales and almost all of them live within 10 miles of the Sydney AIDS Clinic. Unfortunately, Federal AIDS research funding has been decided by using a state by state political formula, rather than on a problem oriented priority basis. Again I assume this reflects community-wide concern as the research has not been directed at evaluating epidemic control programs.

Testing first started in August of 1984 at Saint Vincent's hospital in Sydney using the immunofluorescence technique in a cell line we got from Jay Levy in San Francisco. At that time we were screening about 150 people each week at outpatient clinics and through a number of collaborating general practitioners. In Australia, antibody tests are not done through private pathology services. The government has designated a number of hospital based reference laboratories where initial ELISA screening is done. All positive tests are sent to the main state reference laboratory for confirmation by western blot or immunofluorescence before patients are given their results. All positive tests in New South Wales have been through the Saint Vincent's Hospital laboratory and their accompanying demographic data has been most valuable in assessing the pattern of this disease. When we consider the number of people screened around Australia it is clear again that this epidemic is centered in Sydney. Over 20 percent of the tests performed there are confirmed antibody positive and we estimate that there may be between 35 and 50,000 seropositive homosexual or bisexual men in the state. From this data we could expect the number of end-stage AIDS cases to be higher at this time. It's worth taking a moment to consider whether the progression rate in Australia may be slower than in the United States. I will cover this in more depth in a moment, but two recent observations have some bearing. First, that hemophiliacs are progressing to the end-stage of the disease at a much slower rate than gay men. Second, Jay Levy's workers in San Francisco have found that the AIDS virus is not present in the peripheral blood of 50 percent of asymptomatic antibody positive men, thus showing that they have been able to switch off viral reproduction. It is possible that by making changes in sexual practices, alcohol and drug intake, reducing stress and minimizing exposures that activate T-cell function and therefore virus production, an individual may be able to alter the course of the infection. Data we have gathered in Sydney on a group of more than 3.000 homosexual men indicate that they have fewer overall T-cell stimulating risk factors than do gay men in San Francisco and New York City. Thus, we may be seeing a slower and hopefully lower progression rate of the infection in Australia's east coast cities. Discovering which factors are most important in determining outcome is, in my opinion, our highest research priority. The problem is figuring just how to do this as quickly as possible and convincingly enough, so that early diagnosis of infection becomes a medical issue and not only a social, legal or philosophical debate. It is with this concept of surviving infection with the AIDS virus that I will now briefly outline how the Sydney AIDS Clinic operates as an integrated model of clinical service and research.

This clinic is a free service funded by the New South Wales Health Department. There are now 20 full time or part time health workers and more than 150 volunteers who contribute immeasurably to the clinic. At an average cost of less than $50.00 a visit, we are able to provide a full range of AIDS related services to people at all stages of infection. Because the clinic is free and not based at a hospital, there is no need to collect any definitive identifying information on any person who attends. Therefore, until a patient requires hospitalization their management is totally anonymous. I might add here that our follow-up rate is over 85 percent, meaning that almost everybody comes back for their appointments and we have no need to trace them. The clinic produces educational material and the staff give innumerable lectures. Two activities I will spend some time on later are the evaluation and policy implications of the work we do. But I should just reiterate that the clinic is an early diagnosis and management service for people who do not yet require inpatient hospital care. One of the major concerns of people who are at risk of infection, especially homosexual and bisexual men, intravenous drug users and prostitutes, is that some judicial authority will gain access to their records and because these are identifiable, any admission of illegal activities will be used against them. Some of the best designed epidemiologic prospective studies have foundered because this fear has not been convincingly allayed and because clinical care was seen as separate from participation in research projects. Our first line in establishing a sense of personal security is that we do not collect any names or addresses and do not require confirmation of identity. Each person is given a number which is cross-referenced to their first name, date of birth and zip code, and these are only used if a number is forgotten or lost. All tests are ordered using this number and all data that are computerized are entered with this code. Many of our patients who have been coming to the clinic regularly for a year, and in some cases have become volunteers, do so in the knowledge that their identities and therefore their privacy is assured. A similar situation happened in the United States with the alternate test sites. I feel that their promise of anonymity attracts many people. However, they are neither a clinical management nor a research service and therefore their usefulness in reducing the impact of AIDS is still to be evaluated. To summarize, when a person becomes a clinic client their first contact is with a system that has been set up to meet their needs, and therefore they are generally open to provide detailed and accurate information on important epidemiological behavioral parameters. Each person is assessed by a medical practitioner who collects a comprehensive history of exposure, risk factors, signs and symptoms and life style. We do T-cell subsets on all antibody positive persons and all high risk symptomatic seronegatives. These are repeated every

three to six months depending on disease progression and T-4
numbers have provided the most important prognostic indicator of
patient health. It is our impression that until T-4 numbers drop
below about 150 there is little correlation between signs and
symptoms: typically diarrhea, fevers, weight loss, lymphadenopathy
and immunologic status.

Table 1 compares the symptomatic and asymptomatic antibody
positive men with respect to selected immunological parameters.
There is no significant difference between the groups in any of the
measures we regard as indicators of active AIDS virus infection.
We are also conducting detailed neuropsychological testing on a
sample of well seropositive persons to try and determine how early
brain damage may occur. Again this is an area where research and
clinical programs will need to integrate on a continuing basis.
All data from the clinic are recorded in medical records and each
day the records are computerized. We have done this since we've
started and now have comprehensive information on more than 12,000
patient visits. Thus research, if we can call it that, may be
conducted on a large cohort of patients who can be selected on
clinical or behavioral criteria. For example, if you want to
select a cohort of seropositive men who have a particular set of
signs or symptoms, we are able to select the cases from the
computer, mark their records, and at the next visit they can be
asked to give more detailed information especially about lifestyle
or behavioral patterns. In 12 months we have screened about 4,500
persons. The vast majority of people we see are male. About 60
percent are homosexual or bisexual and 38 percent are
heterosexual. These data are interesting because they indicate
that the clinic is accessible and used by a broad spectrum of the
community. At present we average 100 to 150 new patients each week
and a total visit number of between 400 and 450 patients a week.

Table 1.  SASG Prospective Study

|  | ARV AB POS | | |
|---|---|---|---|
|  | SYMPTOMATIC | SYMPTOMLESS | SIG |
|  | $2 \pm 3.2$ | $3.3 \pm 4$ | P |
|  | N = 170 | N = 183 | |
| LYMPHOCYTE COUNT | $2000 \pm 780$ | $1900 \pm 540$ | NS |
| T4$\pm$ % | $26 \pm 780$ | $29 \pm 10$ | <0.02 |
| T4$\pm$ NO | $510 \pm 300$ | $540 \pm 240$ | NS |
| T8$\pm$ NO | $570 \pm 300$ | $520 \pm 260$ | NS |
| T4$\pm$sTS+ | $1.00 \pm 0.57$ | $1.20 \pm 0.67$ | <0.001 |

Table 2 shows the numbers of new homosexual and bisexual
clients by month since we opened. October and November last year
were two months when media coverage about AIDS was particularly
hysterical. Many of you may have heard of the infant who lived
just north of Sydney and was refused schooling and the family was
ostracized by the local community because she had AIDS. This
publicity seemed to stimulate increased clinic attendance. During
the first 10 months an average of 24 percent of these homosexual
men each month were confirmed seropositive. During the past three
months that proportion has risen to 30 percent. The numbers of
bisexual men have remained remarkable constant. Either they don't
take much notice of the publicity or different factors influence
their seeking screening. Most bisexual men are married and many
have children, so the implications of a seropositive result are
even more frightening for them. An important research question in

this respect is, "What motivates people to be screened?" We try to
get all high risk antibody negative persons to come back every
three months for a repeat test, as we believe this gives them an
added incentive to remain uninfected. The seroconversion rate
among regular clinic clients is less than half of the three percent
we have observed in a separate perspective study of 950 homosexual
men. It indicates that early diagnosis or screening may be an
important co-factor in altering sexual behavior and in reducing
transmission.

Table 2.  Sexual Preference

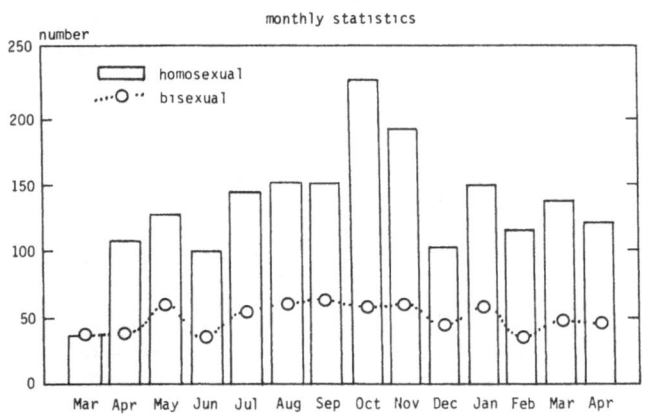

Table 3 shows the distribution of other risk factors among
clients and incorporates many of the females we see. It indicates
that the clinic is not only used by one particular risk group and
there are substantial numbers of people in each cohort to evaluate
infection risk and disease outcome in a standardized clinical
setting. I should say here that the figures may give the
impression that there is constant harmony among patient groups. It
is unnecessary for me to tell you that AIDS is a nightmare of fear
and politics. The organizations that have mushroomed in recent
years to champion and protect their flock from AIDS, all chastise
the clinic, generally in unison, that services and support are not
adequate or appropriate for their constituency. I've come to
realize that the clinic, like all AIDS clinics and wards all over
the world are like the "Grim Reaper," appearing years before
expected and providing a tangible focus for the unlimited fear and
frustration felt by young people who are becoming progressively ill
and dying. Overall, about 12 percent of all people screened are
confirmed seropositive. The proportion, of course, varies between
risk groups.

Table 3.  Client Characteristics

|  | N= | % |
|---|---|---|
| I V DRUG USERS | 432 | 10 |
| TRANSFUSION RECIPIENTS | 375 | 9 |
| PROSTITUTES (MALE & FEMALE) | 163 | 4 |
| PROSTITUTES CONTACTS | 710 | 16 |

Table 4 shows the distribution of risk factors among
the seropositive persons we have diagnosed at the clinic.  In
addition to these we manage several hundred more who have been
referred by local doctors or hospitals, particularly for ongoing
counseling and support.  Because the clinic, in many instances,
provides primary medical care for these people, we have a good
opportunity to observe the natural history of the AIDS virus from
the earliest exposure.  By repeating T-cell subsets and
immunoglobulins on a regular basis we may be able to build an
integrated model of physical as well as immunological consequences
of infection.  Two observations we have made are that T-4 numbers
can vary as much as 70 to 80 percent from visit to visit.  And that
in some individuals a significant and progressive improvement in
T-4 numbers can follow changes in lifestyle and behavior patterns.
Whether this improvement will remain over a long period is still to
be determined, however we have not yet analyzed this data against
controlled seropositive subjects who remain in a fast lane
existence and therefore the observations are really just
anecdotal.  Nevertheless our counseling and support services for
seropositive people are very much directed at providing
constructive programs to help people maximize their chances for
survival and minimize their risks of further infection or of
transmitting the virus to others.  As with many AIDS services our
counselors are young and identify closely with their patients.

Table 4.  Selected Characteristics of Persons Screened
by Antibody Status 1985/86

| Ab+ve | N= | % |
|---|---|---|
| MALE | 520 | 98 |
| FEMALE | 8 | 2 |
| HOMOSEXUAL | 452 | 85 |
| BISEXUAL | 54 | 10 |
| I V DRUG USERS | 51 | 10 |
| BLOOD RECIPIENTS | 29 | 5 |
| PROSTITUTES | 22 | 4 |
| TOTAL | 533 | |

Before leaving the activities of the clinic there are two
services I'd like to briefly mention.  First, the volunteer
services which include the Ankali Project.  Ankali is an Aboriginal
word meaning friend.  It is modeled directly on the excellent
program, the Shanti Project, in San Francisco.  And the hot line,
which is run by volunteers who have answered more than a thousand
inquiry calls each week since it was set up eight months ago.
Because these services are integrated into the day-to-day
functioning of the clinic they benefit from its medical, counseling
and technical support especially as an information reference
center.  And the regular clinic staff benefit from feedback
provided by the widest spectrum of AIDS related experience.  The
hot line is able to quantify the numbers and characteristics of
persons who phone for information, and the Ankali Project is able
to become involved in emotional support care for people with AIDS
as soon as a diagnosis is confirmed, usually after months of
following the same individual through routine clinical management.

The last aspect is one I regard as most interesting.  It has
long concerned me that western medicine has become too
institutionalized.  We sit in our offices and wait for sick or

worried people to come in seeking help.  While that is all right for socially acceptable diseases, AIDS has introduced a new dimension to this practice.  Six months ago we began an outreach program to diagnose and prevent AIDs virus infection among the vast groups of young, disaffected people who would not come to any medical service unless they were at death's door.  I'm referring to the street-based population in Sydney who are at risk for infection.  Each night a well equipped van parks on the streets in heart of Kings Cross in the inner city area and from 9:00 p.m. to 7:00 a.m. a young nurse and counselor take blood for antibody testing and provide information and counseling and condoms to the street kids.  They also visit male and female brothels to talk to their workers about safer sex practices and to assess any AIDS related medical problems.  In a short time the bus has become a focal point for male prostitutes and IV drug users who now have a caring service on their own turf.  As a surveillance research unit the data collected by the outreach project has been invaluable in tracking spread of the AIDS virus among a previously inaccessible population.

Earlier I said I would discuss evaluation and policy implications of the clinic's activities.  A major consideration in evaluating our clinical observation is assessment, compared to those who don't.  I can't really answer that.  There just doesn't seem to be any good baseline demographic data on the characteristics of any of the risk groups, not only in Australia but anywhere else.  Even so, as all prospective epidemiologic studies in AIDS are volunteer based and therefore attract a self-selected population, the data gathered at the clinic is probably as useful as an enrolled cohort.  We have been very careful not to generalize any of our observations to homosexual men or all intravenous drug users.  But in terms of policy advice our data provides public health planners, researchers and clinicians with a readily available data base, on a continually increasing cohort of at-risk and infected persons.  In addition, we have the facility to establish large scale clinical trials for therapeutic agents that may be useful if given early enough in the disease process.

Before concluding, I would like to address the proposal for establishing an international research council.  While there seems to be productive collaboration between laboratory based researchers in most countries and internationally, there is very little cross-cooperation between researchers involved in describing the epidemiological and behavioral determinance of disease progression.  A research council could have the specific brief of designating sentinel clinical units in different countries where standardized clinical management, data collection instruments could be used to provide a comprehensive picture of this epidemic.  It should be technically feasible to establish computer links between centers, to facilitate aggregated data analysis and easy communication.  I would hesitate to suggest that any major research finding should be vetoed by a committee but premature announcements of research finding, especially about clinical trials, have caused our AIDS treatment services untold problems in trying to scientifically interpret short, general press releases for the local media and for hundreds of outpatients who telephone within days of any new announcement.

In summary, there are three issues that we need to address in AIDS research. First, because of the well understood complexities of the AIDS issue, we must adapt our established structures of design and clinical service to both accommodate the fears of those exposed and to enable the medical profession, charged with the responsibility of treating disease, to evaluate the effectiveness of early diagnosis and intervention. Second, public policy decision makers internationally need to realize that this epidemic is in different time frames in different countries and that there are important lessons to be learned. In different countries research programs could be tried and applied in areas where in other countries, like in the United States, they can't be done at this time. And lastly, unless we establish a positive, sympathetic program for research on an international scale, it may be impossible to test any vaccine or treatment that would be developed in the future. Thank you very much.


COMMENTS


Morris Abram, J.D. (Former Chairman of the President's Commission on the Study of Medical Ethics, Vice Chairman, Civil Rights Commission)

Dr. Walters, Dr. Gold, Dr. Wyngaarden, fellow panelists and friends. I may have a slightly different approach than some of the speakers you've heard, because first of all, though I have spent a long time now with the ethical problems in medicine I certainly do not pretend to be an expert on the subject that you're grappling with. Long ago I learned, as a young kid in Fitzgerald, Georgia where I grew up, deep in south Georgia, not to pose as an expert. The days in which I was in grammar school were days of prohibition and we were visited annually by a woman from the Women's Christian Temperance Union to tell us about the evils of alcohol. One day, when I was in the third grade, eight years old - I don't know why I needed to be told or any of us needed to be told about alcohol at that age - but we were visited by this woman who wanted to be known as an expert and she said she was. She was so introduced. She took a glass of water, and she took a glass of alcohol, and she took an earthworm and dropped it in the glass of what she said was water and held up the wiggly, happy earthworm for us all to see and said, "Now, I'll take this worm and I drop it in the glass of alcohol" and she held up the fried, dead worm - very unhappy worm - for us to see. And she looked at us, and with a look of great self-satisfaction and achievement - this expert said "Now children, what does that prove?" Well, one Georgia cracker, in the back of the room, stood up and said, "Woman, that proves that if you've got worms, you better drink whiskey." I am not an expert, but I'd like to introduce a few notes which perhaps have been sounded, perhaps not. Looked at from the viewpoint of the ethical problems of medicine, the problems of AIDS to society, wherever it occurs, present in very stark form the choice between the principle of human autonomy, or the human will, or the human desire, or the human preference, as a way of life and as a rule of society; as opposed to utilitarian system which in effect says that we try to provide the greatest good for the greatest number, and the individual preference and autonomy is subservient to that. I think it is a measure of our society, a barometer of the health of our

society, and its decency that we have not treated the problem of
AIDS with a utilitarian response. We have very much treated it as
a problem, as we should have, involving human autonomy, human
respect. We have not placed people on ice flows, we have not
isolated people as lepers and consequently, I think we can take
some degree of self-congratulation though quite honestly we face
terrible problems which no one must deny. But the problems arise
also in the context of modern society. And it's paradigmatic, I
think, this disease, and maybe other diseases will erupt by virtue
of the kind of society we live in.

Here is a disease thought to have originated in Central Africa,
then transmitted from one place to another, and it's even gone as
far as down under as Australia and it will continue, I suppose, to
multiply and to grow wherever human beings do, to travel, as they
are able, by airplane and every other kind of conveyance. It is a
disease perhaps as a result of some mutation. And God knows how
the mutation was caused. By environmental factors? Human
intervention? God knows. But apparently some of the factors about
this disease arise out of the nature of the international society
and the openness of our experience and the oneness of our
civilization. It also arises, and it presents serious problems, in
the context of human freedom. And freedom is something we value
very, very highly and we would not want to transform the nature of
our society, simply in order to deal with a dreadful disease. Now
there's been a lot of self-flagellation about our countries'
efforts with repect to the dealing with this disease. I say
self-flagellation because I try to take on a historic backward
look, as we have struggled with other diseases in the past, and
compare the progress against this disease with the progress in
other instances. It was a very long time before Edward Jenner
discovered that cowpox could vaccinate against smallpox. It was a
very long time before Koch discovered the universal tubercule
bacilli. It was in almost my own lifetime that by human
experimentation of a rather crude nature, the etiology of yellow
fever was discovered and a long time later there came a vaccine.
We're still struggling with a lot of diseases that do not yield to
modern invention and to modern technique. But since 1981 in the
case of this disease, as horrible as it is the etiology of it has
been discovered and the virus has been isolated. We are told by
Dr. Wyngaarden that the complete deciphering of the genetic code
has been accomplished. We know how it is transmitted. We know
also, which is very important, how it is not transmitted, thus
stilling an awful lot of fear and preventing an awful lot of
panic. Not only that, we can screen human blood so that we can
continue to minister to people who need it. But we have an
extremely tough issue. The Presidential Commission dealt
extensively with the question of human experimentation with respect
to the treatment or therapy for disease. I suppose with this
disease, and to be very crude about it, I imagine there won't be
many difficulties in getting volunteers for human experimentation.
I say that from some personal experience, because in 1973 I was
diagnosed as having acute myelogenous leukemia. I can tell you
quite frankly, they could have done anything with my consent, my
informed consent. Because the choice was between doing something
drastic - dreadful, or death. Consequently, the normal restraints
on human experimentation and consent will not be very difficult
with this disease in its present characteristic. On the other
hand, if you turn to the issue of whether or not if we're able to
find something that looks like a vaccine, whether or not we can

test it, it is going to be damn difficult.  Because a person who does not have the disease makes some kind of admission in asking to be vaccinated and there will be reluctance about it.  And moreover, one does not really know whether or not one has come in contact with the disease after one has been vaccinated.  So the control mechanism is out of kilter.  So even if we do come very close to a vaccine, it's going to be extremely difficult to test it, to say nothing of the problems of liability in testing a vaccine for a disease as deadly as this.

Now, I'd like to deal with just a few of the issues that came out of these extraordinary papers that we've just listened to.  First of all, I listened very carefully to Dr. Wyngaarden who said something that fascinated me.  Perhaps it's because I am a layman.  He said, "In Australia a higher fraction of AIDS cases arise from blood transfusions while there are very few cases as a result of IV drug use."  This is an example of how international cooperation and experience in a vacuum in various places may contribute to the total body of learning.  "It's an intriguing thing", he said.  And I suppose that investigators will dwell upon it, for it may have some significance.  Dr. Wyngaarden also asked, "Why", of, "Is there an unexplained difference in the rate of disease in those African versus those of Asian descent in Trinidad?  Is there some clue here?"  We wouldn't know unless there had been some kind of record keeping or some kind of epidemiologic studies in Trinidad.  Then you see Dr. Gold's paper.  He pointed out, quite correctly, I think that Australia could be seen as an experimental model as yet unaffected by the terrible toll that AIDS has taken on its victims and health workers alike elsewhere.  Well, it's an interesting point that, "Ninety-eight percent of the cases in Australia involve males."  Now, we can all understand why there would be a significantly greater number of males.  But I was intrigued.  And perhaps some of you who are more qualified than I would wonder why only two percent females in Australia.  And how does that compare to the figures in the United States?  And if these figures are disparate, why are they disparate?  What does it tell us, either about the nature of the transmission of the disease, or the nature of the societies?  Dr. Gold also said that he has experienced in his clinic the altering of the course of the infection after diagnosis of the antibody's existence, by change in lifestyle.  That was to me an astounding statement.  Here you've got evidence of a seropositive nature with respect to a deadly disease, the progression of which is thought to be inevitable and inexorable.  He says that there is an altering of the course of the infection by a change in lifestyle.  That has enormous implications.  Then he said something else which I thought was terribly significant to an international body.  He said that in the case of those who are high risk who come into his clinic, he urges them to come in every three months, even when they are negative.  And I got from his paper, the strong indication that that imposed a discipline upon these "prone" persons to remain negative by whatever means.  Almost like Weight Watchers in which you are afraid to come in and tell your guru that you've gained weight.  Powerful psychological weapon in the hands of skillful practitioners and sensitive people.  So I've learned a lot from listening to this survey of experience with this terrible disease around the world.  I close by simply noting that as the Hastings Report said in an issue dealing with this disease, I think about a year ago, "It's not going to be resolved in the way that a cholera epidemic in Great Britain, or England, or London was solved a hundred years ago when a man named John Snow figured that the cholera was issuing from a water pump in the City of London. He stopped the epidemic by taking the handle off the pump." I don't think we're going to yield up sexual practices as rapidly.

Andrew Moss, M.D. (Adjunct Assistant Professor, Department of Epidemiology and International Health, University of California, San Francisco)

I'm one of the lucky people that received funding for AIDS research back in 1982 when the National Cancer Institute issued the first RFP. In 1982 and 1983, it was extremely difficult to get funding for AIDS research from any source, and the process of getting it seemed irrational. Primarily, this difficulty was due to the fact that AIDS was perceived as a homosexual disease. It was extremely difficult for funding agencies, foundations and local governments to deal with the fact that what we had here was a homosexual epidemic.

My experience with the funding system in this country is that it's a bureaucracy. It knows how to do certain things. Diseases have constituencies and these constituencies are organized on a seniority basis, and it's easy to decide who gets money to do what. When AIDS came on the clinical scene in this country, nobody knew whose disease it was. It began with dermatologists, it moved to oncologists then to immunologists and then to infectious disease physicians. AIDS still doesn't really reside in a disease specialty, the way most organized diseases do in this country.

The reason why it is such a nightmare to get money for AIDS research is due to the competitive research system in the United States.

Going back to 1982 - we, in San Francisco, have one medical school - when the RFP was issued by the National Cancer Institute in July of that year, we submitted a proposal. One submission for San Francisco. In New York and the surrounding area there are, I believe, nine medical institutions, and all nine of them submitted proposals also. And as those of you on the research side know, when this kind of thing happens, you withdraw into your own little cell. You cut off communications with people in the same field, because they have become the competition. You end up with nine rotten proposals, and none of them got funded. No one in New York City received funding that year.

As a result, four years later, there was still no dedicated AIDS virology laboratory in New York City. One has been established over the last several months. And New York City had about a third of all the AIDS patients in the United States.

This incident was due, in part, to the competitive pathology of the federal funding system in this country. Science, in this country, is an ego-driven system, and this has become increasingly true with AIDS. With the advent of the bio-technology companies, it is also profit driven as well as ego-driven.

I'm not going to say that this doesn't work. There are some fields of endeavor where this type of system works very well. The ego-driven system encourages very smart people to take their laboratories and work them very hard - sometimes. But there are areas where this doesn't work.

When you have a public health crisis, like AIDS, an infectious disease, a disease of homosexual men, a new disease, you can't rely upon existing mechanisms to work, and you certainly can't rely upon a competitive funding system to work.

I think this is worth bearing in mind, now that AIDS has become an international disease - now that we can think about AIDS in an international perspective.

Although I'm a foreigner, I've worked in the American research system for the last decade. What I have tried to do is to follow the planning committees' recommendations and think about what I would like to see an imaginary, wise, international AIDS coordinating body accomplish.

First of all, I would like to see it change the image of the disease. I think the worst thing that AIDS has suffered from is the stigmatization of the populations - primarily the fact that three quarters of the cases are homosexual men. This prevailing fact has made it difficult for people to think about it. Particularly to think about the public health aspect of it and to come to grips with the changing behavior. I think if we look at AIDS from the international perspective - and we learned this morning from Dr. Clumeck's presentations that African AIDS appears to be a widespread heterosexual disease in Central and Western Africa with blood donor studies showing seropositivity rates between 4 and 18 percent. That is two or three orders of magnitude higher than in this country. That is a terrifying phenomenon. When we look at AIDS in the international perspective, we're seeing not a homosexual disease, but a venereal disease. Primarily a venereal disease, and a disease which is very much a third world disease.

I'd like to see this international body begin to think about AIDS as a North/South problem, in the same sense that debt, international debt, is a North/South problem. In other words, the resources available to deal with AIDS are North. They are in the United States, in Western Europe, Japan and other industrialized countries. The problem is likely to be, I think, increasingly South, in the third world countries, already in Africa.

We should begin to think about what's going to happen in the rest of the third world, and what it means if AIDS spreads at the same rate everywhere else, as it has in Africa. I think the way this would change our perspective on AIDS is that we'd begin to think of it the same way we think about malaria, schistosomiasis and smallpox. It's a huge worldwide problem, not particular to homosexual men. The developed countries have a moral responsibility to attack it on a worldwide basis.

Secondly, I'd like to see this imaginary, international body, present a research agenda to the United States and the other industrialized countries where technology, money and science prevail. This would be a particular agenda, developed to fill a gap.

Right now, we have two very rapidly advancing main fronts of research. The first one is to develop a vaccine and the second one, which is not so fast, but slowly expanding, to conduct therapeutic trials in AIDS. These are both essentially profit driven goals.

They emerge from the fact that there is a well-oiled mechanism for conducting drug trials for sick people in this country, because drug companies make it easy to do. The same is really true about vaccine development. Vaccine development is relatively easy. There are a lot of technology companies who are interested in vaccines.

Both of these are good things, but there is no comparable driving force between a third area, prevention. We need to learn to deal with and treat AIDS early, to understand the carrier state, to understand the mechanism which appears to make some people immune, and appears to put some people in the position of not shedding the virus. In our own studies, we have found that about 10% of highly exposed people never get infected. We find about the same proportion of people who are infected and don't become sicker. There are things going on with this virus that have to do with infection, the carrier state, immunity, which we don't know about and need to explore further. The prognosis for the vaccine, as everybody has stated, is not good, at least not in the next few years. And when I talk to my clinical colleagues, they are uniformly pessimistic about therapeutic trials. I don't believe we will see a miracle drug or a miracle vaccine in the next few years. That makes it that much more critical that we try to intervene elsewhere. Unfortunately, this hypothetical research agenda is very expensive. If the United States or any other western government is really serious about trying to characterize the carrier state and AIDS, and intervene early, then a great deal of money will have to be expended on top of vaccine development and on top of therapy.

If I were a member of this envisioned international body, those would be my priorities. Maybe this isn't a Manhattan Project or maybe it's not an Apollo Project, but it is critically important. It will require tremendous financial resources and central coordination.

I think there are some concrete negotiations that need to take place now, some of which may be taking place already in other countries, which can be useful to us here - reversing the process. Dr. Gold has talked aboout Sydney and one of the things they have done there is used the screening test very aggressively, as a public health measure. In fact, they've screened about 30-40 thousand people in Sydney, as many as have been screened in the United States. What are the effects of this? Why don't we know?

If the United States government is really interested in AIDS prevention, why doesn't anyone go over to Sydney and study their situation and evaluate it's usefulness in this country. It has to be done in Sydney, because people in this country are afraid to use the screening tests as a public health tool. So let's find out how it works when it's used in countries which will do it. Another example of this - along the same lines is free needles. You cannot legalize use here. It's politically impossible. It's been brought up in many jurisdictions, and uniformly gets squelched by mayors or attorney generals or police chiefs. But, you can do it in Europe, it's being done in Holland. They have an evaluated program in which addicts trade in old needles for clean needles, and it's being run by Dr. Al Curtino in Amsterdam. Other variants have been proposed for other European cities.

We could go there and look at them and find out how it works. If it's found to be successful, we can come back and fill a huge gap in our own public policy discussions about this issue here. This idea of central coordination internationally would help us gain access to these alternate methods.

Finally, some thoughts on a vaccine for AIDS. In San Francisco, seronegative homosexual men are now seroconverting at a rate of between 3 and 4% a year, a falling rate. By the time a vaccine is developed, they will not be seroconverting at a rate allowing vaccine usefulness. I don't think that the vaccine will be tested on homosexual men. I would not like to be in the position of testing it on intravenous drug users. As you know, they are a difficult group to follow. Who will it be tested on? I suspect it's going to be tested in Africa. The politics of vaccine use are terrifying in the sense that there is already massive distrust among some African countries of the motives of the western technological countries. If a vaccine is to be tested there, they will respond with - "This is a commercial product for you - You're testing it here. We're taking the risk. What kind of a deal is that?"

I think that we're faced with some very long term and difficult negotiations on the public health side of AIDS. We are in need of a international negotiating or exchange mechanism which is capable of proceeding in a way that's credible to all parties. Thank you.

### John Seale, M.D., M.R.C.P. (Venereologist, London, England)

I would like to put forward a few thoughts as a background to this afternoon session, rather than to comment directly on what has already been said. I speak as a clinician who has specialized in sexually transmitted diseases for over 20 years.

There are some basic, simple, scientific and historical facts underlying the AIDS epidemic which need to be clearly stated and understood if there is to be effective cooperation in dealing with AIDS within individual nations let alone at an international level.

The continued use of the term, Acquired Immune Deficiency Syndrome, is causing endless confusion to the public, the media, politicians and physicians. It was narrowly defined by Centers for Disease Control in mid-1982 for the limited, but specific, purpose of epidemiological analysis of a new disease phenomenon in mankind of unknown cause first described in 1981. The virus causing the disease was isolated in 1983, and by early 1984 the scientific evidence that this virus was the cause of the syndrome was conclusive. Nevertheless, the original definition of AIDS, with only minor modifications, has been retained by CDC, by the World Health Organization, and by government health departments throughout the world, long after its original purpose had been served. Continued use of the term not only impairs the understanding of scientists and physicians of the nature of the disease caused by the virus, it also hides from the public of all nations the gravity of the threat which mankind now faces.

We are dealing with an infectious disease caused by a specific virus which is no more, and no less complicated or obscure, than several other infectious diseases such as tuberculosis, or syphilis, or the manifestations of infection with Beta-hemolytic streptococci. It only seems to be particularly complex because the disease is so new and our technical means of investigating it are so sophisticated. CDC-defined AIDS however, is still essentially a clinical definition of disease in a person independent of any hard scientific evidence of infection of that person with the virus causing the disease. This definition enables governments all over the world to exclude, legitimately, from official statistics, the vast majority of people who are both infected with the virus and infectious to others, and also to exclude the majority of deaths caused by AIDS virus infection.

People who die following infection with the AIDS virus; such death being caused by tuberculosis, bacterial pneumonia, malaria or bacterial dysentery, all of which are common in poorer countries, do not die from "CDC-defined AIDS", even though the AIDS virus may have been grown from their blood and they were profoundly immune deficient. People who die from encephalopathy or myelopathy where the AIDS virus has been grown from their brain, spinal cord and cerebro-spinal fluid, do not have "CDC-defined AIDS" unless they also have infection with some obscure opportunistic microbe which was irrelevant as a cause of death.

Clearly a new infectious disease caused by a new virus must have a name. For simplicity, I shall call it "aids" spelled in lower case letters. This is how the intelligent public describes the disease. Whenever I refer to those late manifestations of the disease covered by the now rather archaic official definition, I shall call that "CDC-defined AIDS".

Once we are clear what we are talking about, it becomes easier to define the nature of the problem about which cooperation is required at national and international levels. Here are some key aspects of the problem which are often missed, or just fudged.

"aids" is the first entirely new, highly lethal, specific viral disease to emerge as a worldwide epidemic spreading from person to person, since the foundation of the science of microbiology. The epidemic spread started only in the late 1970s. It is a problem with which modern medicine has no previous experience.

"aids" has the essential characteristics of a slow virus disease. That is, there is an incubation period normally lasting several years, and sometimes many years, during which the person is clinically well, but potentially infectious, followed by slowly progressive disease from which there is no permanent recovery.

Within five years of infection with the "aids" virus, whether through contaminated blood transfusion, contaminated clotting factor, shared hypodermics or male homosexual activities, about 25 percent of infected people in the U.S.A. have developed "CDC-defined AIDS". Consequently, "aids" is already known to be one of the most deadly viral infections of humans, far more deadly than infection with the Lassa fever virus and more so than smallpox virus. What the ultimate mortality will be for individuals 20 years after infection nobody can yet know. There are, however, viral infections in man and animals where mortality, following infection, regularly exceeds 90 percent. Rabies in man, maedi-visna in sheep, which has so many similarities to "aids" in man, and malignant catarrhal fever in cattle.

The "aids" virus causes persistent or intermittent viremia and is characteristically blood transmitted, rather than sexually transmitted. Consequently, the virus is spread most rapidly by

58

repeatedly reused, unsterilized hypodermics, whether by intravenous drug addicts in New York or in Edinburgh where over 50 percent are already infected, or medically reused hypodermics in third world countries, the Soviet Union and east Europe. Sexual manuevers that damage the rectal mucosa of people who frequently change partners transmits the virus far more rapidly than orthodox sexual practices, as with other persistently viremic diseases such as Hepatitis B.

Once a critical mass of people has been infected by highly efficient means of transmitting the virus, then transmission by far less efficient means will inevitably occur increasingly often. These include blood transfusion, perinatal transmission, biologically normal sexual intercourse, needle stick injuries, chance contact with sores or abrasions with blood, perhaps mechanical transmission by blood sucking insects and routine dental procedures.

With serial passage of the "aids" virus through the human population, evolutionary pressures of natural selection will favor those genetically determined strains of the virus which are most readily transmissible. Consequently it is probable that the "aids" virus will become increasingly infectious as the pandemic evolves.

This is just some of the important background of what I perceive to be the reality against which national and international cooperation is required.


Susan Zolla-Pazner, Ph.D., (Co-Director, AIDS Center, Manhattan VA Medical Center)

One of the issues that we have been addressing is whether our glass is half empty or half full. One example of this is the 150 million dollars, approximately, that's been devoted to the study of AIDS this year. I think it's perceived outside of this room that 150 million dollars is a lot of money. I think it's perceived within this room and by people who are involved in the study of AIDS that 150 million dollars is not a lot of money. For instance, even with this money only a very small percentage of individuals who want to be included in clinical trials are going to be included in those trials. Even with 150 million dollars, certainly nowhere near enough money is being committed to public education. So that even with 150 million dollars committed for spending on AIDS this fiscal year we have insufficient money for just these two efforts. This leads me to two more issues: the effect of this restricted support on developing information about the pathogenesis of AIDS and the effect of this shortage of funds on deterring collaboration and fostering competition. In addressing the first of these issues, I want to address what is not being done or not being done sufficiently, in my view, with this money. One of the speakers this morning mentioned that politically attractive solutions are not necessarily philosophically correct. I'd like to point out that politically attractive solutions are not necessarily scientifically correct. It is not as popular to support basic research as it is to support applied research. It is much easier for the public to grasp and understand attempts to develop drugs, attempts to develop vaccines, than it is for the public to understand efforts to, for instance, understand some of the complexities of the immune response to HIV or the complexities of the genetic structure of the virus.

I have to ask, however, whether it's correct to spend millions and millions of dollars on drug development programs, on clinical trials, and on vaccine development without simultaneously underpinning these efforts with aggressive programs in basic research that eventually are going to be applicable to this disease. Let me give you an example: We are trying desperately to develop a vaccine to this virus in the absence of knowledge about the body's protective response to it, thus, the vast majority of individuals who are infected with HIV are healthy at this time, asymptomatic and living in balance, at least for the time being, with this infection. Is this due to their antibody response to this virus? We don't know. Is this due to the ability of their lymphocytes and other lymphoid cells to constrain the growth of this virus? We don't know. Is the humoral antibody response more important than the cell-mediated immune response? We don't know. Look at it from the other perspective. The vast majority of patients who have ARC and who have AIDS have antibodies to the virus and yet most of the antibodies that are circulating in the blood of these patients are not neutralizing antibodies. They do nothing, as far as we know, to impede the growth of this virus in these individuals. Look, if you will, at the beautiful cover of today's program and you will see a computerized model of a perfectly healthy virus to which three antibody molecules are attached. It does not show a virus particle which is coated with antibody, engulfed by a macrophage and destroyed. We don't know yet enough about the basic mechanisms of the body's ability to immunologically handle this disease. I give these examples, not because they are the only examples, but because they are the ones that I am most familiar with as an immunologist. And so I use this as an example of the point that I want to make: that it is nearly impossible to develop a vaccine in an intelligent and rational way in the absence of this absolutely basic knowledge about how the immune system handles this infection. Yet, very little money is being spent on the basic research that will give us the information to develop such a vaccine.

As an example of how little money is being devoted to basic studies of AIDS, last year the NIH supported one RFA (request for applications), to support studies on the immunologic mechanisms at the basis of HIV infection. That RFA was advertised as providing a total of 1.5 million dollars for the support of immunologic studies. 1.5 million dollars is only one percent of the 150 million dollars that's been committed to AIDS and only enough to support three or four projects over three years, hardly a substantial commitment to basic AIDS research.

I remind you of something that I think all of you know. It is certainly a commitment in the past that NIH has adhered to strictly, that you must go to the lab before you can go to the bedside. Certainly we couldn't have isolated and identified HTLV-III if we hadn't first identified T-cell growth factor. The basic studies are the foundation for the applied studies. Therefore, at the international, the national, the state, and the private level we have to look for greater commitment for basic studies on this disease. It is not a popular alternative, but it is one that's absolutely necessary.

If there's one consensus that I've heard this morning, it is the pessimism of almost everybody in this room that we are not going to have, probably, a magic bullet in the next 10 years in the form of either a drug or a vaccine. If that gloomy prediction holds true, then certainly that is another reason to support this aggressive commitment to basic research that will help us deal with this disease. It is important to consider the effects of the shortage of funds on competition within the medical and scientific community. Obviously, where there's a shortage of funds there's going to be competition. The competition I have to say, is not as bad in the AIDS field as I think it is in many other fields of medical science. And indeed I've seen more collaboration and more effective collaboration amongst researchers working on AIDS than I've seen in nearly 20 years in medical research. But "publish or perish" still prevails. It is often very difficult to enlist the participation of individuals in large collaborative studies for if one group shares its data with another group and the second group publishes with first authorship, then ultimately the first group may be relinquishing their ability to get funds down the line. So there is indeed competition between individuals who are doing work on AIDS. In addition, there is competition between the individuals who are doing work on AIDS and those biomedical scientists in other areas who are resentful of the set aside money that is being devoted to AIDS. It is therefore creating a certain amount of friction within the system itself, and one that needs to be addressed.

Finally, I want to mention that in the absence of sufficient public funds to support some of this research, a number of scientists are turning to the private sector. Indeed this is something that's being fostered by the present administration. While there are advantages to this, there are also disadvantages. One example that I could give is of a conversation I had several months ago with an excellent scientist, who is working on the structure of the HIV virus. When I asked certain specific questions regarding the structure of the envelope protein of the virus and the sequence work that he had been doing, I was informed that he couldn't give me that information. That the information, in fact, would not be soon published because the information would go first to the private company that was supporting the research. As a result, the private support, the scientific community in general was being deprived of information. And in the long run the results are going to be slow to get out and slow to be developed. So this shortage of funds is affecting our efforts at all levels to move on this disease.

I ask, therefore, not for you just to send money, but to send it in an intelligent way, a way that is chanelled not from a politically motivated point of view, but from a scientifically sound point of view. I ask that the expenditures be made with a view to the long run and not simply the political short run. Thank you.

Keynote Address:  AIDS:  A Classical Public Health Problem in
Modern Guise

Frederick Robbins, M.D.
Former President, Institute of Medicine, National Academy of
Sciences

KEYNOTE ADDRESS:  AIDS: A CLASSICAL PUBLIC HEALTH PROBLEM IN MODERN

GUISE


Frederick Robbins, M.D.

Former President, Institute of Medicine
National Academy of Sciences


It's very difficult to talk on the subject of AIDS.  I can't
think of anything that's more talked about these days.  To say
anything new is almost beyond thinking.

No occurrence in recent times has generated the degree of public
concern, scientific activity and puzzlement among public health
officials than what has come to be recognized as the pandemic of
AIDS.

The seriousness of this problem was not immediately recognized
widely.  Although it was a highly fatal disease, the number of cases
was small.  It affected special populations (male homosexuals and
intravenous drug users) whose plight did not necessarily evoke great
sympathy in the general population.  Indeed, certain persons made
statements to the effect that AIDS was a punishment God was
inflicting upon the sinners.  Therefore, righteous need have no fear.

This attitude soon lost its credibility when it was found that
the disease could be transmitted by transfusions and contaminated
blood products such as Factor 8 used to treat hemophilia.  Obviously
the problem was more widespread.  With the identification of the
etiologic virus and the development of laboratory techniques capable
of identifying infected individuals, the scope of the problem in the
United States became truly alarming even to those more complacent or
skeptical.

The last threat to public health of comparable magnitude was
probably the influenza pandemic of 1918 and 1919.  However, the two
events are fundamentally different in that the flu epidemic was
sudden in its onset, involved a large proportion of the population
in a brief period of time and ended abruptly.  This is clearly not
true of AIDS.  It's most impressive, I think, to recognize how much
we have learned about AIDS in a brief period of about five years.
This has been possible, above all, because of the knowledge gained
and the techniques developed in basic molecular biology, immunolgy
and, of course, the special study of retroviruses.  This point was
made very vividly yesterday by Dr. Wyngaarden, but I'd like to
reemphasize it.

I know of no better example than the importance of a strong basic science program, and the pay-off that this can have in solving important practical problems, often totally unanticipated. In a brief period the causative agent has been identified, tests for the identification of infected individuals have been developed and much progress has been made in elucidating the pathogenesis of the disease. Also, much has been learned about its epidemiology and significant progress has been made towards a vaccine. While a great deal remains to be done, and even though there have been complaints that the government did not move quickly enough nor apply adequate resources to deal with AIDS, one cannot help but be impressed with the progress that has been made.

Another aspect of the AIDS situation worth noting is the great importance of international cooperation and what has been learned from studies in other countries, particularly Africa. Once again, it is brought home to us that disease is no respecter of geographic or national boundaries. Scientific expertise is not limited in any particular country and the language of science is universal. Unfortunately, those of us in science, public health and medical care, who are so acutely aware of these facts, have not communicated this message very effectively to the general public nor to the majority of responsible policy setters in government.

I would like to suggest that AIDS presents society with a public health dilemma which requires answering a series of classical questions that are no different for AIDS than for polio, measles, syphilis, or Legionnaire's disease. However, AIDS has occurred at a time when we have the powerful tools of molecular biology which were not available only a few years ago. Therefore the approach to the problem can be quite different than was the case with many diseases in the past.

From what we know about AIDS, it seems to me that we have to approach it both from the point of view of the treatment of the disease and its prevention. We all recognize that there is no satisfactory treatment for AIDS and not very good treatment for the opportunistic infections which so often are the cause of morbidity and mortality. Anti-viral substances are being developed for a variety of viruses and a number are being tested for efficacy against AIDS. The retroviruses, with their integration into the cell gene, present a particularly difficult problem. Theoretically, it should be possible to develop the means to prevent the activation of the provirus and prevent the presence of infectious virus in the blood. We need to understand the factors involved in activation. These are areas we don't understand too clearly. Treatment directed at maintaining the latent state is more likely to be successful than treatment directed at eliminating the integrated genome. That's a tough prospect. However, it does suggest that treatment may have to be maintained for life.

In spite of the lack of specific therapy for AIDS, patients require a great deal of medical care and psychological support. In communities such as New York and San Francisco, AIDS care places a major burden on the health care system at all levels. The cost of this care stresses an already over-burdened system and if we feel over-burdened in this country, think of the situation in a developing world. This situation, at least temporarily, will get worse. One of the very important policy questions that federal, state and community governments are going to have to consider is how to apportion resources to deal with this question. I can't help but comment that it would be easier to have a universal health insurance or something similar.

In turning to prevention there are two aspects to the prevention of AIDS. First is prevention of infection with the AIDS virus. The second is prevention of overt disease. This is not different from many other situations. In polio, the vaccine prevents disease; it doesn't always prevent infection. There is a distinction. There are various ways of preventing a disease which include the epidemiological approach, in which various means are employed to interrupt transmission based on the knowledge of its epidemiology, and artificially enhancing a resistance to infection by passive or active means.

At the moment the epidemiologic approach is the only way we have to deal with the problem. We do know enough to accomplish a great deal if we put it to practice, provided the concerned persons can be persuaded voluntarily, or if necessary by coercion, to modify their behavior. Some of the measures that can be recommended must be based on the fact that this is a venereal disease and sexual practices, whether by male homosexuals or heterosexuals need to be reduced in amount and to some extent degree. Monogomy is clearly the best policy. There is a great deal of talk about the need for safe sexual practices. As far as I know, the only safe sexual practice is achieved through the use of the condom, and we all know that this isn't always as successful as we would like it to be.

The question of protecting the blood supply has been talked about at length and I think we can say that a great deal of progress has been made. It is not 100 percent. Even though test results are very good, they still have a three to five percent error rate. There is always the possibility that the person is infected but has not yet expressed antibody so there continues to be the possibility of some slippage. The statement that we have 100 percent safe blood supply is not, in my opinion, sustainable. While the rate is very good, it does mean that the use of transfusion must be thought about, and should not be done without some consideration of the risk benefit ratio. This is particularly relevant to the parts of the developing world where the administration of blood is done for what we consider quite unnecessary reasons. If and when a test for antigen is developed then this might help close that small gap.

The issue of syringes and needles is a difficult one. The use of common needles and syringes is dangerous. The major population at risk in this country is the intravenous drug user. This is a particularly difficult population to reach. From the epidemiologic point of view, and this is particularly true in New York these days, this is a critical group since they spread infection to their mates and are probably responsible for many of the neonatal infections. As repugnant as the idea may be to many people, it seems to me that the time has come to seriously consider providing needles and syringes to drug users to avoid the necessity of using common instruments. Whether this will work in the United States I don't know. It seems to me worth considering as a demonstration. Also we have to reconsider, in some communities at least, the methadone situation. I know all the problems with methadone, but it would be a way to assist in curtailing AIDS transmission through sharing needles.

In the developing world, the situation is quite different than it is here. They do not control their use of blood as well as we do. The multiple use of syringes and needles is quite common in vaccination programs and in therapy. They do a lot of injection. In fact, in some countries, therapy is not regarded as effective unless it is given by needle. Pills are seen as having no use. Some people feel that in parts of the developing world, transfusions and the improper use of syringes and needles are a major means of AIDS transmission.

There are things that can be done to prevent infection but much of it depends upon changing personal behavior. This is never easy to achieve, but in view of the alternative, if people truly understand the situation, many will respond and indeed have. However, in order to attain maximum response it will require an intensive, imaginative, educational campaign. Admittedly there are very special problems of societal prejudice towards the gay community and the need to maintain confidentiality is particularly important with this population. Furthermore, sexual practices are particularly difficult to change. However, the drug users will probably be the most difficult group to reach.

Little is known about how to prevent the occurrence of overt disease, among those already infected. Some recommend total abstinence and the adoption of a healthy lifestyle, whatever that may be. There are no data that I know of to really document the efficacy of such a program even though it has its adherents and strong believers and I see no likelihood that it would do harm.

Enhancing resistance is primarily being approached through efforts to develop a vaccine for active immunization. It seems somewhat unlikely that passive immunization, that is, introduction of antibody, will be effective where the virus is so intimately associated with the cell. However, in the absence of precise knowledge of the events that occur at the time of infection, one cannot be sure that an antibody passively administered would not protect. It seems to me that it would be worth a try in conditions of particularly high risk. I understand that a trial is being developed in this country.

In order to develop an effective vaccine it would be important to know which of the antigens associated with the viral particle are responsible for stimulating immunity or protection. Indeed, it is not certain that antibodies are protective at all. Much attention is being devoted to the envelope protein which because of its location on the surface of the virion seems the most likely target. This protein happens to be the element most subject to variation. Whether or not this is significant from the point of view of protection is not known. Unfortunately the lack of a suitable experimental animal is a serious handicap. The rhesus monkey may prove to be a useful model but whether it provides a model for humans is still not clear.

One may be forced to test for the presence of infection, that is actual virus isolation tests, in order to prove the effectiveness of the vaccine. That certainly would very much complicate the assessment of a vaccine. Most likely the first vaccine to be available will be composed of one or more of the protein subunits of the virion. Techniques have been developed for the production of the antigens by cloning, which has obvious advantages over the use of the whole virus. When an experimental vaccine is ready for testing in humans there will be the problem of selecting a suitable population for assessing efficacy. The population has to be cooperative, and of sufficient size with a rate of new infections and disease that is statistically significant. There are not any such groups available. Indeed, to assess the impact on disease when the incubation period may be two to five years clearly presents a major problem.

This is not the place to discuss all that is required in order to prove that a vaccine is safe and efficacious. However, there is no doubt that testing potential vaccines against AIDS poses special problems, and although progress to this point has been most gratifying, there are yet many obstacles to be overcome and one should not expect a generally available vaccine licensed as safe and effective for some years.

So far, I've spoken only of inactive vaccines. Other alternatives are being considered which include live attenuated vaccine and vaccinia virus as a vector for the AIDS virus antigen. The idea of the use of attenuated strain has been stimulated by the recent isolation of asymptomatic persons in Africa of a strain of HIV which is closely related to the simian viruses. This might turn out to be a useful approach but only after an intense study of the epidemiology of the infection and the characteristics of the agent. One would hesitate a long time before deliberately inoculating normal persons with an agent having the properties of HIV virus. Use of the vaccinia virus as a vector has certain appeal. The molecular biology involved in introducing foreign genes that are expressed into the genome of the virus is an elegant science and may prove useful in other situation. However, in view of the serious reactions that have occurred in the virus of immune deficient individuals, one would be very hesitant to vaccinate those in high risk categories, some of whom might already be infected and suffer from varying degrees of T-cell deficiency.

Indeed I understand that the army had one case of disseminated vaccinia in an immunodeficient person who was vaccinated. It's interesting to speculate on what one would do with a licensed vaccine if we had it. The high risk population would be an obvious target. However, in the U.S. these consist of mainly homosexuals and drug abusers and the latter group would probably be difficult to reach with a vaccine or anything else. The homosexual population might well be quite responsive. However, whether that's a large enough population to attract the attention of commercial manufacturers, I don't know. If not, it might be necessary to subsidize the production of the vaccine.

Another population that might be considered is the military. I have no idea how great the problem is in the military, but if the risk were great enough a vaccination might be useful.

A matter of some concern that needs elucidation is what would be the result of vaccinating those who are already infected with the antibody. Will the vaccine enhance protection of re-infection or superinfection if such occurs? Will it simply have no significant effect or will it serve as an antigenic stimulus and provoke viral release in occurrence of overt disease that seems to occur in the test tube? We don't know the answer to that.

Some people have suggested that maybe an AIDS vaccine might be one administered generally with the routine immunization program. This seems to me quite unlikely and probably quite unnecessary. However, in some developing countries it might be considered.

Thus, in summary, it seems to me that we have the tools to develop a vaccine from the laboratory point of view. Testing of this vaccine and exactly how it would be used still present unsolved problems that I see as major impediments to the quick introduction of vaccination as a major solution to our problem.

In the broad policy arena, there are two major issues remaining. One is a chronic one, the allocation of resources. AIDS has required decisions in regard to research, support of clinical care and education. New money has been made available for AIDS research, some of it by the states most affected and some has been diverted from other areas. The results have been very gratifying but again I'll point out that they would not have been nearly so effective had there not been available the results of years of basic research in immunology, retrovirology and molecular genetics. This was made possible by other policy decisions to support biomedical science. Although the resources devoted to AIDS necessarily divert funds from other purposes the research being conducted will add to our knowledge in cell biology, immunology and other areas. So it's not wasted.

When considering how funds allocated for AIDS should be apportioned, it would seem important that education receive a very high priority since it is the foundation for the epidemiologic method of control, and the only means that we have available at this time. This may well be true for a number of years to come.

Underlying the whole AIDS issue is the common public health problem. Namely the rights of the individual as opposed to the welfare to society as a whole. In our society we give priority to the rights of the individual except in exceptional circumstances. For instance, we legally mandate children be immunized in certain diseases in order to be allowed to enter school. This is coercion. In the case of AIDS this dilemma is accentuated by the desire of many to avoid being identified, largely because of the prejudice of many in society.

It seems to me that legislation, which you may hear about later, recently passed in Sweden is a model worth looking at. This requires that anyone that has reason to suspect that they might be infected with HIV contact a physician who can confirm or disprove infection and if infection is demonstrated, provide social and psychological support. Infected persons are enjoined to take measures to prevent spreading of the disease by sexual intercourse, they are forbidden to give blood, mother's milk, organ transplants, sperm for insemination or to pass on to someone else a hypodermic needle he or she has used. They are also required to inform health personnel of the potential risk to them in dealing with blood products from the person in question. Safeguards are taken to maintain confidentiality, including special coded system for the laboratory tests. Up to this point, everything is voluntary. They do provide compulsory measures including enforced isolation, if other means have failed. This seems a rational approach that makes every effort to protect the individual, but in the last analysis, the needs of the community must prevail.

70

One hopes are that a society that really understands the issues will react responsibly. However, societal members must be given the facts in a straightforward manner. The credibility of authority is not high in this country at this time, and every effort must be made to avoid the appearance of propaganda. So far, in spite of some overreaction from where I sit, it would appear that things have been more tranquil than one might have expected. Perhaps the obvious pace of scientific advance has given the public a sense of the problem being approached appropriately. A constant danger is over-promising. Personally, I recoil when statements are made that we can expect a vaccine in two years, when I know what a complicated problem it is to develop any vaccine and realize that a vaccine against AIDS presents more difficulties than most. We have a serious problem on our hands. There are some things we can do now and we are dealing with some of them reasonably well.

For the future, we have no alternative but to place our faith in the ability of science, whether molecular or epidemiologic, to provide the answer. Societal mechanisms will then have to be put in place to put the discoveries in practice. In some ways this is the most difficult part of the process.

A great deal of the success of the program in this country will depend on our public health departments. They have not been well supported in recent years, in fact, more than just recent years. New York and California are reasonably fortunate in having pretty effective departments. Many of our other states do not. I think it's time that the public realized the importance of public health and support those who are trying to protect our health in the same way they support those who are doing those dramatic things in the operating room.

Session C: Clinical Management: Treatment Modes and Impact on the Health Care Systems

Participants

Speakers

David Axelrod, M.D.
Commissioner, New York State Department of Health

Mervyn Silverman, M.D., M.P.H.
Health Care Consultant, Former Commissioner of Health, City and County of San Francisco

Panelists

James Curran, M.D., M.P.H.
Director, AIDS Branch, Centers for Disease Control

Donald Abrams, M.D.
Assistant Director, AIDS Activities, San Francisco General Hospital

Michael Adler, M.D.
Chairman, Department of Genito-urinary Medicine, Middlesex Hospital Medical School, London, England

Sheldon Landesman, M.D.
Associate Professor of Medicine, Director, AIDS Study Group, State University of New York, Downstate Medical Center

Eric Sandstrom, M.D., Ph.D.
Associate Professor, Department of Dermatology-Venereology, Karolinska Institute, Stockholm, Sweden, Secretary, Swedish Government Delegation on AIDS

CLINICAL MANAGEMENT:  TREATMENT MODES AND IMPACT ON THE HEALTH CARE

SYSTEM

James Curran, M.D., M.P.H.[1],
David Axelrod, M.D.[2], and
Mervyn Silverman, M.D., M.P.H.[3]

INTRODUCTION


### Dr. Curran

Let me just mention a couple reflections now that we are close
to our fifth anniversary of the first report of AIDS and three years
since the evidence that a retrovirus caused the illness (first
laboratory evidence).  It's probably about four years since most
people were pretty sure that it was caused by an infectious agent.
It's been two years since the majority of the scientific world
believed that it was due to an HIV infection and fifteen months
since the licensing of the serologic tests.  New York City and New
York State have really played leadership roles in the recognition of
virtually every stage of the problem and the entire world has often
looked to New York and the United States for ways to deal with the
very complex issues related to AIDS.

There are now 21,000 cases reported to CDC from 50 states, the
District of Columbia and three territories with estimates of a
million or more persons with HIV infection in the United States.
Cases have been reported from 80 to 90 countries with cases
diagnosed in residents of over 105 countries of the world.  So AIDS
is an international, global problem.  We are no longer dealing with
a problem that is going to be entirely solved soon, if ever.  What
does`that really mean?  The problem is here in New York City and
it's been here since 1978 or so.  It's a chronic, endemic disease
problem that has to be dealt with as a chronic disease problem.  The
first cases of AIDS in the United States, and perhaps in the world,
were recognized in New York and California and in New York City the
first cases were recognized in intravenous drug users, heterosexual
partners, and spouses.  The first cases in pediatric patients were
recognized in New York, cases of prisoners were recognized in New
York, and some of the first cases in transfusion recipients in

---
[1]  Director, AIDS Branch, Centers for Disease Control
[2]  Commissioner, New York State Department of Health  [3]  Health
Care Consultant, Former Commissioner of Health, City and County
of San Francisco

Haitians were recognized in New York. Everyone has looked to New York in recognition of the problem and is now looking to New York and the United States for solid long term solutions of what is essentially a chronic disease problem as well as an acute infectious disease problem.

You have an opportunity this morning to advise us. We represent not only the federal government, but the state government, private foundations, clinicians, etc. I'd like you to think about what you would have us do if we had an extra $100 million, $200 million, $300 million in taxpayer money, be it state taxpayers, city or federal taxpayers. What would you do and what kind of accountability would you demand for that money? How would you prove the money had been spent efficaciously?

Secondly, I'd like you to think what you want the country to look like vis-a-vis AIDS 1990 or the year 2000 if there is no vaccine or no therapy. I think it's most useful for those of us who are not molecular biologists and aren't involved in anti-viral therapy to think of what will happen in the absence of vaccine or therapy. First, I want to minimize the number of persons infected with the virus. To me that is paramount. Secondly, I want to maintain civil liberties. I don't want our society to be ripped apart. But first I want fewer people infected with the virus. I want fewer people infected with the virus.

Let's think about this as a chronic disease problem, a chronic health problem. Think about what we have to do to solve a chronic health problem and what kind of approaches we need. First, planning is necessary. This is not something that is going to be solved by individuals in any kind of isolation with solutions that are devised overnight. Secondly, put time in some perspective. What we do today isn't as important as what we have done over the next three to four years. So when you are thinking about issues of serologic testing and thinking about issues of testing and counseling, civil liberty issues, let's have solutions that we can live with three or four years from now. Let's make sure that if we are using serologic tests we do everything we can to make sure they are used appropriately while maintaining civil liberties. Finally, let's have commitment, let's have solutions that involve things like five- or ten-year budgets, not just one-year budgets.

Our first speaker has been introduced before and many of you know him. To me he represents the very best kind of person we can have in public health. A distinguished scientist, someone who has demonstrated public concern for health problems and a capable and effective administrator, Dr. David Axelrod.


DISCUSSION


### Dr. Axelrod

I'm a little bit uncomfortable talking about the management of a problem after it has occurred as opposed to providing for a refocus on some of the initiatives that might have prevented the disease in the first place. The concerns that were voiced by Dr. Robbins, I think, are shared by all of us in public health. The concerns focus on a lack of support and an erosion in fact, of the resources that would provide for additional preventive activities, educational efforts, and all of the things that go along with the traditional approaches to public health. For those who have viewed the public health scene historically, you are aware of the fact that the major advances with respect to public health have come about not as a result of cures, not as a result of forms of surgery or major advances in technology, but rather with respect to some of the sanitary initiatives that have characterized the public health process in the United States and so many other countries. I'm a little sensitive, therefore, in talking about the ways in which New York State has managed the problem of dealing with a disease after it has occurred as opposed to providing for additional preventive measures.

However, in the absence of a vaccine and the absence of effective therapies, states like New York have a responsibility for governmental initiatives that demonstrate their social responsiveness, their concern, and their ability to provide for those who are afflicted with the disease. Dr. Curran has made a very telling point with respect to an organization that is going to provide care to these individuals in the years to come. When we talk about the care and treatment of individuals who are afflicted with AIDS we address them not from the perspective of today but rather from the perspective of what the problem is likely to be in two or three or five years with some form of therapeutic approach, with some expectation of perhaps a vaccine, but also with the knowledge that there may not be the cures on the horizon that we are looking for. There may not be effective therapies. There may not be effective vaccines for dealing with the problems confronting us. So, in looking at the whole of the planning process, we must develop several different scenarios to deal with the critical problems that we may face in the future.

New York State as part of its response, has established an AIDS Institute that assumes all of the responsibilities for coordinating services, educational and preventive activities, in dealing with AIDS in the State of New York. The AIDS Institute is within the Department of Health. Our concern is that there be a coordinated effort, an entity that brings together all of the services that are part of an overall initiative to deal with the crises we are facing at the present time.

For those of you who are not familiar with the New York State medical system, you should be aware that we have both eleemosynary and governmental institutions that are part of the health care system. We do not have a large number of the so-called entrepreneurial institutions that are direct providers of health care. We do have, in New York City, the largest group of municipal hospitals anywhere in the country. I think it is important to recognize that these public hospitals are a critical part of the health care system and have represented a course of last resort for a large number of individuals. So, we have a very diverse system of care.

The major concern we have had with respect to the clinical management of patients is that there be equity of access to health care. We believe that there is an entitlement which exists for all individuals, and that they should have access to high quality health care. Another concern that we have had is that patient concerns and comfort should be paramount; they transcend provider needs and concerns.

In looking at the ability of New York State to provide for the care of those individuals, a number of things became immediately apparent. First of all, there was an enormous concern on the part of health care workers themselves in dealing with those individuals that were known to be infected with AIDS. As a result of a major educational effort and cooperation with virtually every sector of the health care industry, we have effectively dispelled some of the initial concerns that did in fact interfere with access to health care for those with AIDS. We have continued this major educational process to assure that those who are coming into the health care system are aware of the facts as we know them today about the transmission of HIV, the origin of the disease itself, the progress of the disease and something of the problems that are likely to be faced in the care of those individuals. Unfortunately, the problem of dealing with large numbers of cases of AIDS came at a time when there was a revolution in health care reimbursement. Institutional providers, because of the changes in reimbursement systems, were very much concerned with the impact of caring for individuals who required high intensity services. We in New York State have had a prospective reimbursement system for some time, although it has not been a DRG-based system. It has been a cost-based system that is designed to encourage the efficient production of health care services. At the same time as we were trying to assure access to health care, institutions were becoming very much concerned with the cost of the services to this group of individuals who required a higher than normal intensity of health care.

Another major concern related to the populations with which we were dealing was the different support systems and the different spectra of illnesses. The spectra of illnesses that were identified in the IV drug user population were somewhat different from that which we saw in the homosexual population. The number of cases of Kaposi's sarcoma, and the kinds of secondary infections that occurred were distinct. In many cases, the IV drug user population represented a larger liability to the provider institutions than did those within the homosexual population. What began to appear was a process by which those who were most acutely ill and who did not have the kind of financial support systems existing within the homosexual community began to end up in the municipal hospitals and the governmental system and those who had such support systems ended up within the voluntary system. So we had a division, and continue to have some division with respect to the provision of health care services based not necessarily on the severity of illness, but on purely social and economic considerations.

Additionally, we are especially concerned with the needs of children. Those of you who have followed the discussions here are aware of the fact that we have a disproportionate number of children with AIDS in New York State as compared to the rest of the country, and in comparison to the total number of AIDS cases. This is related to the fact that we have a disproportionate number of IV drug users with AIDS. These IV drug abusers and their sexual partners have been the source of a large number of children who have come down with AIDS and this problem promises to be a continuing cause of concern here in New York State.

Another major interest was to assure that there was a research focus and a comparative study ability. As we looked at the numbers of cases in New York State and the problems relating to the evaluation of care, we were determined to build into the system a means of evaluating the effectiveness of the therapy, or therapies, employed. This was a major element of the way in which we organized health care services.

Finally, as we evaluated what was happening with respect to the care of the patients, we also became increasingly concerned with the special needs of those with neurologic disease. The ability of many institutions to care for individuals who were neurologically impaired was often quite different from their ability to deal with the usual acute characteristics of AIDS as it was originally defined. So what we were faced with was the organization of health care services in a fashion permitting us to address the problems of access, patient needs, and at the same time deal with the concerns of the health care provider community. We also needed to assure ourselves that we had established a process by which we could conduct comparative studies that could ultimately lead to major advances with respect to the treatment and, possibly, the prevention of AIDS.

The difficulty, of course, is that there are conflicting incentives in every part of the health care system. Our first concern was that we should eliminate barriers that related to reimbursement and to determine, in fact, what the differences were with respect to the costs of the care for those patients with AIDS as opposed to others cared for within the health care system. As a result of our own studies as well as the study carried out by the Greater New York Hospital Association, it became clear that the costs associated with the care of patients with AIDS was approximately 20 percent higher than care for the average person within our acute care institutions. As a result of this information we have provided for an increase in reimbursement to those institutions that care for substantial numbers of AIDS patients.

We also have recognized that there was a need for a case management system. The initial cases in New York State were largely within the homosexual community (the gay community) and they had organized a very effective system of personal support systems. As we began to see additional cases occurring within the IV drug population, we became concerned with the fragility of the personal support systems that were available to those afflicted with AIDS. It became increasingly clear that we needed to have a comprehensive management system to deal with each individual patient. There needed to be a recognition of the personal and social, as well as medical needs of these individuals.

We recognized that in many instances the nature of services is dictated by the available revenues. The availability in our system of services to the AIDS community was very much based upon who was going to reimburse for what medical services. Many of the services that are reimbursed are only those that provide direct medical services and not the kinds of social support systems that are absolutely essential to the continued care of individuals with AIDS.

As a result of these discoveries we determined that we should have a series of centers within the state of New York to provide for the full component of AIDS services. In January of this year the New York State Hospital Review and Planning Council, which is the formal body that approves changes of health care services, adopted emergency measures to amend the public health law to designate certain hospitals to be centers for the care of AIDS patients and authorized the Commissioner of Health to approve applicants who might wish to be involved in the comprehensive care of AIDS patients. The goal of the system of the designated centers is to permit patients to maintain the quality of their lives in a home environment as long as possible. The centers will provide or arrange for all levels of care and services required by AIDS patients, including ambulatory and in-patient services, home care and personal health care services, psychosocial and psychiatric services, arrangements for needed housing, legal and financial assistance, and appropriate hospice and residential health care services. It is important to note that voluntary organizations in New York State had, for a very long period of time, assumed the responsibility for the provision of many of these services. The voluntary systems were being overwhelmed by the addition of new cases of AIDS and no longer able to deal with the additional problems of the increasing numbers of children, the increasing numbers of individuals from the IV drug community. This comprehensive responsibility for a wide range of health and non-health services is to be implemented through a case management model and the centers are to be responsible for the development of a comprehensive management plan for each patient cared for within these centers.

A multidisciplinary team is responsible for all aspects of a patient's in-hospital and post-hospital needs and a case manager is assigned responsibility for coordinating the service needs of each patient to ensure that specific service needs are identified and fulfilled.

We anticipate that as of two months from now, 15 hospitals will become designated AIDS centers in New York State in 1986. The hospitals as part of the system will receive a higher reimbursement for each patient. This rate is approximately 20 percent higher than that received for the care of other patients. The goal of the system that we are putting in place is to coordinate services outside the hospital as well as within the hospital, and to keep patients from unnecessary hospitalization. The program, in many ways, is similar to the model of the San Francisco General Hospital, except that everyone, eventually, with AIDS in New York State has the opportunity to be in the system. It is anticipated that there will be no distinction between the services that will be available to every member of the population, whether it be the IV drug user population, or the gay community.

The regulations that have been put in place require that quality assurance efforts be undertaken to monitor and evaluate the quality and appropriateness of AIDS patients by the center through mechanisms which include the evaluation and monitoring of the patient management plans, utilization reviews and quality assurance programs. In addition, we anticipate that the criteria that will be developed to test the effectiveness of the AIDS centers and whose needs are being met by ad hoc establishments and by hospitals which are not part of the formalized AIDS center institutions. The implementation of this program will be a first step in facilitating full access to services, controlling costs, identifying major existing unmet needs, developing a data base and information for further planning in reducing inappropriate utilization of existing resources.

The number of average monthly hospital AIDS admissions in New York State since 1985 was 473, with an average monthly rate of increase in admissions of approximately 3 1/2 percent. The average length of stay in New York State hospitals was 21 days in 1984, although the more recent data show a significant downward trend. In 1984, typical AIDS patients experienced multiple hospital admissions and a median cumulative survival period ranging from 18 to 125 weeks, depending upon the type of opportunistic infection recorded.

While specific cost data for New York patients are not available, the per case medical costs of patients has typically been within the range of $50,000 to $100,000. The medical needs and the costs of the patients with the disease, vary substantially. Major social and psychological variables are characteristics of these groups and require very different treatment modalities.

In addition to those that have case definition of AIDS, there is another large group of individuals who may be taken care of through this very same system, those who have the need for services that are far less extensive than those that are required for patients with clinical AIDS, and that is the so-called ARC population. Hopefully the hospital utilization by the ARC patient will be lessened by the availability of these AIDS centers that we are establishing at the present time.

In the absence of a federal government initiative for the organization of health care for these individuals, the burden is increasingly falling to the states to provide cost effective care. Certainly in the absence of a program, such as the ESRD program, which provides for the entrance of AIDS patients into Medicare without the two-year waiting period, the states are increasingly going to have to bear the cost of services. No matter what the projections are, this will be a major problem for the Medicaid programs of the states that are caring for these individuals. It is unfortunate that we are shielding the Medicare trust fund by virtue of our Medicaid system in those states that are affected, but that appears to be the direction which the federal government has pursued. We have sought to have the waiting period removed for those patients with AIDS but given the current views of the federal government with respect to Medicare, unfortunately I'm not very hopeful that that system is going to change. Our efforts have been directed at finding cost effective utilization, but not to deny patients services as a result of costs that are to be incurred by the care of these individuals. We have a governmental responsibility and I think that we have an obligation to exercise that social responsibility in the most effective way that we can. We believe that in developing the kind of system I have outlined to you, we can provide those services in an effective and efficient fashion and at the same time control the misallocation and misutilization of resources. Given the absence of a national policy to organize and finance the treatment of patients, each state is going to have to develop its own system that provides for an exercise of the responsibility that government ultimately has.

Dr. Silverman

We have over 2,000 cases in San Francisco and more than half have died. The survival is between zero and 60 months, with about a

13-month median.  Of all cases, 50 percent survive less than 12 months.  For 50 percent of the survival time individuals are in fairly good health; 40 percent of that time they are chronically ill and are debilitated and about 10 percent of the time they are in the terminal stages.

There are several basic concepts that we looked at as we started facing this tragic epidemic, at that time we weren't sure exactly what we were facing.  One was that government can't do it all. Knowing that government can't do it all, we certainly didn't expect the community to be the initiator, the planner, and the implementer of all of the programs.  We began with the idea of a cooperative, collaborative arrangement.  In short, a partnership.  If anything is a cornerstone of any success we've had, that is it.  We didn't plan a model.  We didn't sit back and say we're going to develop this thing.  We, in many instances, were reactive.  In some instances we were proactive and I think what developed has become for many a model, but certainly it was not our intention at the time.  We knew that it was a new health crisis needing a new approach.  If there are two things that come out of this tragic epidemic - positive things - they'll be the following.  One is the team approach in the out-patient unit and the in-patient unit.  Under my administration were two hospitals, San Francisco General Hospital and Laguna Honda Hospital; the first a 450 bed acute care hospital, the second a 1200 bed long term care facility.  The problems were there and are still there, and they seem to always revolve around the hierarchial structure between doctor, nurse, messenger, clerk.  I think that it has been this kind of thing that has been detrimental to health care in our country.  The AIDS in-patient and out-patient teams (doctor, nurse, messenger, clerk) in a lateral (parallel) rather than in a hierarchial structure has had a great deal to do with the kind of care, the positive supportive care, and also the interrelationships between health care providers.  I think it's something we ought to see spread throughout the health care system.  The second thing I hope we can see move into the future is the out-patient network. Communities have it all there, although it is in many pieces.  I think what we've been able to do with AIDS in San Francisco, and I think what's being done with AIDS in a number of areas, is put together this community infrastructure, as I call it, providing a continuum of care containing in-home services and various elements working together which allow the patient to move out of the hospital into a more humane setting.  Of course, one of the really good spin-offs in this day and age is reduction of health care costs. There is no reason that it can't work in cancer care, in long term chronic respiratory care and many other chronic conditions.  It certainly doesn't have to be peculiar to AIDS.

In San Francisco, we saw the first cases in 1981, and as they started to increase, they seemed to be localized in the gay community, and in fact the percentages have really not changed with the years.  Approximately 97 to 98 percent of the cases in San Francisco have been and still are in the homosexual and bisexual community.  In '81 when we saw it happening in this community, I already had in place a lesbian-gay coordinating committee in the department because we have a large gay population in San Francisco. They have health care needs and we wanted to meet them in a sensitive, compassionate way, and also make sure that our staff understood the issues.  So this committee was in place and started work right away putting together a resource document for this new disease, describing what it looked like, and where you could get some care.

In 1981 we established a reporting system for AIDS, making it reportable in a registry for AIDS cases. We tried to investigate and interview when possible all of the cases. We established liaisons between the Department of Public Health and the hospitals, private physicians, and the CDC. Jim Curran's office has been, I think, superb in the support that they have given and in the working relations that we have had. I think it's been a symbiotic relationship and really shows how different levels of government can work well together.

In 1982 we established the Multidisciplinary Clinic at San Francisco General Hospital. It is called Ward 86, and you are going to hear from Don Abrams in more detail about this clinic. It really is a multidisciplinary clinic with diagnosis follow-up, education and counseling.

As the number of cases increased, we added screening clinics at city public health centers. The idea was that people could go there and if it looked like this was a case of AIDS, they would then go to the out-patient clinic.

In 1983 I established the AIDS Activity Office and I think that this was very important. What we did in this office was coordinate and link the continuum of services, to try to identify service gaps and develop plans to address them, to oversee, monitor and support AIDS related contract services, to anticipate funding requirements and then try to maintain and where necessary, expand the department's liaisons.

In July of 1983 we opened the first dedicated in-patient ward in the country, and that was a ward of 12 beds within San Francisco General Hospital. I was reluctant when people came to me and asked that we set this up because at that time I was fearful that we would further isolate the patients and would further inculcate, if you will, the whole leper phenomenon you are seeing related to AIDS. Fortunately I was convinced otherwise, and I think it's one of the finest units I've seen anywhere. It integrates that kind of horizontal relationship between the health care providers, that I described earlier. You hear things from the patients like they feel safe, they feel secure, they feel confident. It is really something to see. It is a unit that can't probably be set up (or shouldn't be set up) in every community, but where possible, I think it's a very positive kind of facility. It has now been doubled in size. We still don't have enough beds on that unit and in all frankness, patients that are in other units around the hospital don't receive as good care as they get in the in-patient unit. Everyone who works in that unit volunteered, in fact there were more people asking to work on that unit than there were openings. There has essentially been no attrition and I think that it's absolutely incredible when you think about the psychological pressures that are brought to bear on the health care staff as the result of seeing these young people die. So I think it really speaks to the importance of that team effort.

Also, brought to bear in this unit is counseling and support services. The Shanti Project in San Francisco has a volunteer assigned to each patient, not only for emotional support but also for advocacy to get them through the maze if they need social services or get SSI, or whatever else they need.

We funded counseling services involving both professional and lay practitioners for the people with AIDS. We started a concerted effort in education. Especially important was the cooperation we received from the gay organizations, especially the AIDS Foundation and a number of gay businesses. In the first year we distributed over a half million pieces of literature, predominantly to the gay community, but also to the general population. We found it very important since there are a number of bisexuals with families outside the city who come into the city and have homosexual relations and then go back. We obviously could not reach them through gay publications because they were not going to carry these back to their homes and their neighborhoods, so we tried through the general press to get the information out that we needed to reach this population.

Between 1982 and 1984 we conducted over 500 training sessions, educational programs and forums. We established a hot line and received tens of thousands of calls every year. We put signs in buses, bars and billboards. We did public service announcements on radio and television, some directed to the gay community and others to the general population.

In the summer of 1983, with all of these activities over the last year, we've seen incredible anxiety. I couldn't understand why the anxiety level was so high. Then I woke up one morning and understood why. Here was government saying don't worry. It's the same government that says don't worry about Three Mile Island, etc., and was now saying don't worry about this disease (unfortunately government is considered the same whether it is federal, state or local) the cause of which we don't know, a disease for which there was no cure and no vaccine, and it was universally fatal, but don't worry about it. So we tried to get more information out as best we could to the community. One of the things that was important was establishing an AIDS medical advisory committee, made up of physicians from the medical society, the blood bank, the gay physicians group, various hospitals, the VA and San Francisco General Hospital. If we were going to do anything about this anxiety, one of the things we'd have to do is try to say the same thing, making sure that we were aware of the latest research information, and weren't speaking at cross purposes. Nothing is worse than having physicians and other health care providers getting up and making uninformed statements. The public doesn't know who to really believe and if they hear one physician say something, they assume that it is the considered medical opinion everywhere. I think the classic example of this and how terrible it can be is the three physicians who walked into the Houston City Council prior to the election last November wearing their white coats and stethoscopes, suitably draped, stating that they were clinicians at Baylor. They proceeded to say that the public should be warned not to shake hands with strangers because they could get AIDS from the sweat. They were supporters of the "Straight Slate" and obviously they had an agenda that was quite different than trying to reduce the spread of AIDS. So we have to make sure that the responsible physicians are well informed and know the answers to the questions, and have somewhat of a unified front so we don't add to the anxiety.

We also established an AIDS Advisory Committee from the community and this has worked very well. Today, San Francisco is spending over $9 million. The services that I've mentioned and the ones that I will mention now could not have been accomplished without a responsive legislative, and executive branch of government, and a supportive community. That is another obvious factor that doesn't exist in other communities, especially in more conservative areas. Every request that I took to the mayor was funded almost always at the level requested. The Board of Supervisors were very supportive. We received no negative response for spending this money for this purpose rather than for other perceived needs in the city.

Presently, we do AIDS screening in two locations seeing about 480 patients a year and that represents about 940 visits. Our out-patient clinic is seeing about 1500 patients per month. There are emotional support services, psychological assessment and short term therapy for those on the waiting list for psychological therapy and educational support groups to promote healthiness for people with AIDS.

We have also involved private physicians. We brought them in and got them involved because we were seeing the number of cases in San Francisco General increasing and we didn't want San Francisco General to be an AIDS-only hospital. It is a teaching hospital, a community hospital. We also knew in San Francisco that half the beds were empty in private hospitals and that administrators were more than happy to fill them. They just didn't want to do a lot of talking about it. So what we did was refer patients to private physicians in the community and they would admit patients using the private hospitals. At the present time, San Francisco General is seeing only 35 percent of the cases. The other hospitals, especially Kaiser Hospital, are seeing the remainder.

With regard to extended care services, most are contracted out. We have a contract for four beds with a private hospital and sometimes seven beds are used out of those four beds, so they have expanded them when we've needed them. We also have public health nurses who provide health assessments and referrals for the people with AIDS. They make about 450 visits to about 150 clients per year.

We contracted with Hospice of San Francisco who provides RNs, medical social workers, home health aides in attendance who provide health monitoring in the home. They have a daily case load of about 50.

The AIDS Foundation has an information referral and hot line and is receiving about 2500 calls per month. We have a social service advocacy group through the AIDS Foundation providing case management including assistance in applying for financial aid. It is handling close to 900 clients per year. We also have, through the AIDS Foundation, emergency housing where we lease single family-type residences and we put four to six persons needing emergency shelter. The average stay is two weeks and can last up to two months. This again is very important because a number of people are thrown out by landlords, lovers, and don't have money to support their rent. We also have long term housing. This is run through the Shanti Project. It is low cost, long term housing for displaced people with AIDS. The aim is to provide more than just a shelter. It provides a home-type of environment. We have home health care services provided in these facilities and we now have about 35 rooms in three- and four-bedroom units. In some of these residences, individuals are assessed 25 percent of their current income if they have it. If they don't, it's supported by the department and through private donations.

The Shanti project provides emotional support and this has really been a tremendous program. They provide hospice counseling and information to people with AIDS, families and loved ones, on the issue of death and dying. They have 220 volunteers who have contributed annually over 70,000 hours.

Practical support for daily living, by the Shanti Project, also assists people with AIDS with activities of daily living. This includes transportation to the clinic and to the grocery store. They also go to the store themselves and buy food for people with AIDS, cook the food, sometimes do laundry and other daily chores. They are taking care of about 450 clients, providing about 30,000 hours of service.

The area of substance abuse services is one in which we are just getting involved. We don't have the kind of problems that New York has. The percentage of IV drug abusers ("pure" IV drug abusers) is less than one percent. About 12 to 14 percent of the homosexual, bisexual people with AIDS in San Francisco are drug users. We assist the staff in our substance abuse programs to understand the AIDS issue and to deal with patients in their care to prevent the spread of AIDS.

I wish we could say we had the kind of program that Julian Gold has in Australia. We have a youth outreach program to try to reach the street kids. There are a lot of kids that come to San Francisco and hustle in the streets and really feel that they are invincible. Obviously, they too can catch this disease.

We also have an alternative testing site in the city. I have been encouraging people in high risk groups to take the test in the kind of situation that we have in San Francisco, that is totally anonymous, totally voluntary, and with very intensive counseling. I think it's shown, although we don't have a control group, that there have been statistically significant behavioral changes among those who have tested positive or tested negative, so I think it is a very important service.

Another important program is the AIDS Health Project, which is a large program providing psychological and general health assessments, with special emphasis in dealing with those things that reduce immune function. There are support groups focusing on the prevention of depression and stress and promotion of safe sexual practices. Finally, we also have a large educational program in the range of two million dollars dealing with media advertising, news and features stories. You'll be hearing this afternoon from Jim Bunn who is with KPIX, a television station that has dedicated a team to covering AIDS. This, I think, is very important so that we get good reporting. The responsible reporting of Jim and his staff has been outstanding. I think it has helped both to lessen anxiety and keep the public informed.

We have, as well as KPIX, put out pamphlets and various other material. We still continue to have many educational events and a number of peer support groups. In short, there is a lot of education going on.

The result of all these programs in San Francisco has meant an average cost per patient of about $30,000 and the average length of stay is under 12 days. Of course, it must be taken into consideration the types of patients and everything else. But I think that those concepts applied in any community should help reduce length of stay and provide more humane care. We still have many problems facing us. The surplus the city had and was able to use to fund these things no longer exists. Gramm-Rudman is barreling down on us so the availability of funds is in question, as the number of cases increase.

I want to end by reiterating what is the cornerstone of our program, what appears to be the basis of the New York program and what will have to be of any program that is set up here or any other place in the world and that is the cooperative and collaborative efforts of government and the private sector and to try and deal with this tragic disease that is obviously going to be with us for a long time. I wish all of you luck in the great battle.


COMMENTS


Donald Abrams, M.D. (Assistant Director, AIDS Activities, San Francisco General Hospital)

I would like to expand upon Dr. Silverman's comments, particularly as they relate to what we are doing at San Francisco General Hospital with regards to care of people with AIDS. In San Francisco we experienced a plateau of AIDS cases averaging 64 to 74 new cases each month for 16 months, from October 1984 through January 1986. Suddenly, for reasons that remain unclear, in February 1986 we suffered a huge increase in our cases for that month, jumping to 101 new cases for that short month alone. We hoped that perhaps this increase was going to be an artifact because cases the next month fell. However, in April we were again up to nearly 100 cases of AIDS in San Francisco. Unfortunately, our death toll in April of 1986 was also the highest that we have experienced since the beginning of the epidemic. We now have over two deaths a day from AIDS in San Francisco.

The average age of an AIDS patient in San Francisco is 35 years. Ninety percent of our patients are caucasians, 97 percent are homosexual. The average patient has a college education, one-quarter of the patients have professional degrees above college and the average income of an AIDS patient in San Francisco is $25,000, somewhat above the median for the city as a whole.

As we heard for the situation in Manhattan, AIDS as a cause of death in San Francisco, surpassed the cumulative totals of accidents, homicides, suicides and cancer in years of potential life lost in men age 25 to 44.

We heard from Dr. Silverman about the concerted effort that the city of San Francisco, largely due to its healthy surplus, has been able to mount in the care and studying of the disease in our city. I would like to concentrate on what we have done with regards to the delivery of medical care as well as the conducting of clinical research in the AIDS Activities Division at San Francisco General Hospital.

.San Francisco General Hospital is the city and county hospital which sees all patients in the city regardless of their ability to pay. In 1982, we opened an AIDS clinic devoted entirely to the care of people with AIDS. Currently we have six half-day clinics a week, and we see an average of 1400 patient/visits each month.

In July of 1983 we opened the first of its kind AIDS in-patient facility, a 12-bed unit at San Francisco General Hospital. Under the direction of Dr. Paul Volberding, the philosophy of the AIDS Activities Division has been to provide optimum care for people with the disease in a multidisciplinary fashion. Our professional staff is made up of personnel representing various sub-specialties related to AIDS, including medical oncology, infectious disease, pulmonary and neurology with input also from dermatology, ENT, ophthamology and certainly psychiatry.

Spanning the gap to provide necessary psychosocial support to our patients with AIDS, we have on-site, in both the clinic and in-patient unit, health care providers who deal with the psychosocial problems of our patients - medical social workers, psychiatric social workers and representatives from the community-based agencies, particularly the Shanti Project, to provide counseling. We believe that this coordinated effort between the groups taking care of both the body and the mind of the patient provides optimum care.

The number of AIDS patient hospital discharges in San Francisco continues to rise. San Francisco General sees about 33 to 35 percent of all people with AIDS in the city at this time. Kaiser Hospital, the largest health maintenance organization in the city, sees another 10 to 15 percent. Currently, the majority of patients are seen by the other hospitals in the city. However, we provide services for the largest single quantity of patients in our clinic.

Our original in-patient unit, 5B, was 12 beds. On April 8, we expanded to 5A, which is now a 20-bed unit. Unfortunately, this is already too small. The average number of AIDS patients hospitalized at San Francisco General over the winter has been between 30 and 45 patients. This is on a medical service of 100 patients. That does impact quite a bit on the patient population that our house staff sees.

We believe that locating all of our patients in a central unit has done a lot to coordinate care. The ward nurses have become expert in the AIDS problem. They teach the nurses on the other wards and, in fact, nurses from all over the city and the world, how AIDS nursing care can best be provided. We also believe that having all the AIDS patients on one unit provides a central focus for the very active and strong community-based support that we receive. Rita Rocket, in particular, has become a folk legend in San Francisco. She is a travel agent during the week. Every other Sunday for the past two years, Rita has catered a meal for all of the AIDS patients hospitalized. She serves and provides entertainment during the Sunday brunch. This is just one example. The refrigerator in the patient lounge at San Francisco General's AIDS ward was donated by the San Francisco Police Department, who keeps it loaded with juices for the patients.

A recent headline in the local newspaper claimed "AIDS Forces Doctors to Alter Training". This refers to an article written by one of our senior residents and appeared in the New England Journal of Medicine. The resident was pointing out some of the problems in working in an "AIDS hospital." During the course of his residency he had taken care of more cases of pneumocystis pneumonia than pneumococcal pneumonia. The same resident published another article soon to appear in the American Review of Respiratory Diseases on his work on the utilization of intensive care beds by AIDS patients. Despite the fact that we've had an increasing number of patients admitted to San Francisco General Hospital with AIDS, utilization of the ICU by patients with AIDS and respiratory failure has virtually fallen off. This stems from the knowledge that the survival of patients admitted to the ICU is only 13 percent, and from active counseling of patients regarding intubation versus non-intubation by the house staff, by the physicians, nurses and Shanti counselors on admission. Although changes have occurred in house staff training, the house staff, nave been able to benefit by publishing articles from the unique experiences they have had.

Similarly, we believe that housing all the patients in a single unit provides optimum care and is able to cut down on the costs. We've heard from the CDC that the average cost of care for an AIDS patient is $150,000, in New York it's $50,000 to $100,000, and in San Francisco, as we heard from Dr. Silverman, our average runs about $30,000. We believe that this is due, in part, to the strength of the AIDS activities, both out-patient and in-patient at San Francisco General Hospital as well as the abundance of community based professional and volunteer services.

As also mentioned by Dr. Silverman, the average length of stay of an AIDS patient in San Francisco is now down to 11.9 days for 1985. This again reflects both the strength of the in-patient unit as well as the ready availability of out-patient services on a daily basis in the out-patient clinic at San Francisco General Hospital. We are also able to discharge patients to home perhaps sooner than to other places because we do have a very active community support system. The Visiting Nurse Association as an active unit which sees AIDS patients at home and can continue, in fact, antibiotic or analgesic therapy via intraveneous approaches in the home allowing us to have patients discharged at an earlier date. For those patients who are no longer going to benefit from any therapy, we also have an AIDS hospice. At this point in time there is no physical building, although one of the churches in San Francisco has recently donated a structure that will serve as a physical hospice for 10 patients. Hospice of San Francisco is more of a treatment philosophy and the Hospice of San Francisco has a dedicated AIDS unit of nurses who take care of patients in their homes in their terminal stages.

Only 15 percent of patients admitted to our unit, 5A, expire in the hospital; 85 percent are discharged to their home. Most AIDS patients in San Francisco can now die in their homes.

The Shanti Project, the community-based gay grassroots organization is also very important for providing not only counseling but practical support at home so patients can be discharged to home and with their Shanti volunteer can get help buying groceries, bringing them to clinic, doing housework, etc.

Again, I think the San Francisco General out-patient unit also serves to provide optimal care to our patient population.

Originally, beginning with one doctor, two nurses and a secretary, the AIDS out-patient clinic has expanded. We have a large medical staff. We have our own laboratory with three personnel drawing blood and coding specimens. We have a full-time doctor of pharmacology, psychosocial support staff, a Shanti counselor, a medical social worker and a psychiatric social worker. Andrew Moss' epidemiology program is located in our clinic as is the group studying AIDS women in San Francisco called AWARE (Association of Women AIDS Research and Education).

Very integral to our services has been the development of a clinical trials group which is made up of protocol managers who administer and collect the paper work of patients enrolled in our drug protocols. We also have data managers for entering this data into the computers. Forming the base of our unit is our administrative and clerical staff.

With this group we have been able to perform a large number of clinical trials. We were doing 12 open protocols on patients with AIDS and AIDS-related conditions in the month of March. We have also done studies with biologic response modifiers and anti-virals in treatment of AIDS. Beginning in mid-1982 under the direction of Dr. Volberding, we looked at alpha interferon in three different dosages and routes, followed by gamma interferon, and subsequently the anti-virals suramin and HPA 23. Currently we are entrusting ribovirin and AZT. Each one of these is being heralded as the hoped-for magic bullet and a potential miracle drug.

Having noticed that patients with the AIDS-related complex are at risk to go on and develop AIDS, we have become less reluctant to enter patients in clinical trials as well. Since the middle of 1983 we have examined the efficacy of alpha interferon and isoprinasine and currently we are in the midst of evaluating AZT and ribovirin in patients with AIDS-related conditions. None of these agents has really proven to be truly efficacious. Alpha interferon, the first drug that we began to study in 1982, however, is the only drug which has had any impact on Kaposi's sarcoma lesions. About one-third of patients treated with this substance achieve some response in their Kaposi's sarcoma. Those patients who did respond to alpha interferon seem to be protected from the development of opportunistic infections. We have not demonstrated any benefit on the immune system. These studies were done prior to the point where the AIDS retrovirus had been identified. So we do not know whether in vivo antiviral effect occurred although in vitro alpha interferon has been shown to have anti-retroviral activity.

Similarly, gamma interferon and interleukin-II showed no benefits. Suramin, interestingly, was able to convert 5 of 23 patients to culture negativity. However suramin was quite toxic. Of these five patients who became culture negative for HIV after treatment with suramin, actually all of them but one had progressive disease. What we see with an antiviral, such as suramin, is a microbiologic cure with clinical disease remaining. So the question is, is viral positivity what we should be studying when we look at the effectiveness of these agents?

In conclusion, one of the problems that we have had in our clinic is balancing enthusiasm for the latest drugs with the reality of the situation. The media is very quick to hopefully pick up on something that may or may not be relevant. We had some difficulty in clinic on the day when headlines appeared saying that AIDS vaccine and treatments were in sight. This was Monday, April 21st. On that day in clinic, we had 110 patients with AIDS scheduled in our clinic. I was the attending physician in the afternoon clinic. The clinic was delayed two hours in an effort to explain why this article said that AZT is an effective drug against the AIDS virus, why therefore, are we only treating 10 patients with drugs and 10 with placebo. Why is the placebo study necessary? Why can't everybody who wants AZT get it if it is in fact effective?

I think it's important that we continue to transmit information along the standard routes of scientific literature and a peer review that we have done in the past. As we heard from a recent questioner, we in San Francisco also have a problem with many of our patients very frustrated with our inability to enter them on treatment protocols. There is a very large traffic from San Francisco across the border to buy drugs. We do understand the patients' needs to be doing something and not to passively sit there as this disease destroys them.


**Michael Adler, M.D.** (Chairman, Department of Genito-Urinary Medicine, Middlesex Hospital Medical School, London, England)

The amount of disease that we have seen is very small compared to the amount here in the U.S. In terms of clinical management of patients in the United Kingdom there are really no differences between the U.K. and the U.S.A. There are, however, some differences in terms of the epidemiology and health care system, which I will talk to you about.

There are three areas of difference that I would like to highlight. The first is that we have far fewer cases. The second thing is that proportionately, we have far more cases in homosexual men, 88 percent compared to your 75 percent. Thirdly, we have far fewer cases in drug addicts at this point in time, only about one percent. The male to female ratio in the U.K. is similar to that in the U.S.A.

The seroprevalence in homosexual men at this point in time is lower than in San Francisco and New York. I'm not certain that we have used the American experience to our advantage in the honeymoon period that you gave us.

In 1982 in my own clinic, three percent of asymptomatic homosexual men were seropositive with a five-fold increase over a period of two years, to 21 percent in 1984. It is now 35 percent.

Interestingly in provincial centers outside London, the rate is very low. But even that has doubled between 1984 and 1985 from 5 to 10 percent.

Most of the cases of AIDS have been seen in London. There is definite geographical clustering of AIDS in the U.K.; 75 to 80 percent of cases have, so far, occurred in London.

As I mentioned, the number of cases in drug addicts is very low indeed, only one percent of the total, and you can see that unlike some of the European experience, we don't quite mirror the Italian or the Swiss experience at this point in time, even though there has been a quadrupling between 1984 and 1985 of the prevalence, and we are now at about 10 percent throughout the U.K. There have been pockets of very high prevalence, particularly in Scotland, where the prevalence amongst addicts in the general practice was 50 percent.

The final two groups are prostitutes and hemophiliacs. In the U.K., there has only been one study looking at the prevalence in 50 prostitutes, and the prevalence was zero. France and Italy also show the same in non-drug addicted prostitutes.

Hemophiliacs are the final risk group that we have in the United Kingdom. The national rate of positivity is about 30 to 35 percent. However, there is some geographical variation.

That is the basic epidemiology as it exists in the United Kingdom. Let me tell you a little bit about the clinical system. Many of you will know that we have a national health service in the U.K. which is financed through taxes, but which means, effectively that no one pays a fee at the time of receiving a service from a physician. Health care is not a financial worry for individuals in the U.K., even though as individuals and members of society, many of us would feel that the budgeting for health is not as high as it should be in relation to spending in other areas.

As well as having a national health service, Dr. Curran has alluded to another service of which we are very proud, which is free and confidential service for sexually transmitted diseases. This was a service that was set up in 1916. It was set up in true traditional British fashion following a royal commission, established after the realization that the morbidity associated with the venereal diseases was very high. For example, in the first World War, we know that of the British and allied troops 25 percent suffered from syphilis and gonorrhea and the annual mortality in England from syphilis was about 50,000. So it was a considerable problem. The royal commission suggested setting up a free and confidential service. We think that in the U.K. the majority of people who have overt sexually transmitted disease do go to clinics. They are not managed by private physicians or primary care physicians. There are 230 clinics throughout the U.K. into which people can refer themselves.

I mention the STD service because it has placed us in very good stead with the advent of AIDS. It has meant that we have had clinical staff used to dealing with homosexual men, and hopefully whom homosexual men have trusted over the years and to whom they are now able to turn.

The second thing is that having an STD service in existence has meant the relationships between the clinician and the scientist have been well developed over the last 20 or 30 years. Many of us had been working closely before AIDS came along with virologists and microbiologists so that the interface between clinical work and research has already been there.

How have we tried to control AIDS in the U.K.?

The first thing that we have done, of course, is to try and develop a very good surveillance system. We do have an informal surveillance system, whereby clinicians notify cases to our British equivalent of CDC. AIDS is not a notifiable disease as I mentioned previously, and as I also mentioned, there has been a political move to make it notifiable. Many of us at this point in time defend that it should not be notifiable because of the fear that this will drive it underground.

The second element of control which we have tried to establish in the U.K. is to develop a network of counseling facilities and good health education. The Department of Health has set up an advisory committee, which is chaired by Donald Acheson, and which has brought together physicians and scientists and interested parties to try and coordinate a policy for the United Kingdom. One of the things that the committee realized was the importance of setting up counseling facilities. So three training centers are being set up to provide training for people in counseling. The goal is that every part of the United Kingdom should eventually have people who are able to counsel. These would be people who are not necessarily medical.

The other committee that I should mention is the British Medical Research Council, who have tried to coordinate epidemiological and therapeutic research by getting scientists to work together in a coordinated fashion. Once individual scientists have established their own territory and their own expertise, they are prepared to work together more readily. The Medical Research Council recognizes the need to make people work together. I think that we are entering a phase now of a good and happy cooperation.

Health education is an area that has worried me considerably, because as I mentioned early on, we had about three or four years advance notice from you in America, of how this epidemic was going to develop, about how the seroprevalence was changing in high risk groups. We had the evidence from San Francisco and New York and it seems to me that we missed, and didn't capitalize on that period of warning that you gave. So far the only health education that has been funded by the government is a one-page advert in national newspapers about three or four months ago. At the same time as mounting this newspaper campaign, pamphlets were produced by our health education council which people could send for.

We have not managed yet to grapple with health education or see it as enough of a priority. It seems to me that unless we can provide extensive and appropriate health education in provincial centers in the U.K., we will see the same level of prevalence as we have seen in London. In the United Kingdom the best health education, the most imaginative health education has in fact, come from the voluntary sector, and particularly the Terrence Higgins Trust. I am very honored to be associated with that Trust and to be a Director. They have not only addressed health education to gay men, but also now to intravenous drug addicts which is not being taken on by the government so far, and also prostitutes.

The third arm of control is obviously screening and I don't want to go into that in great detail. All blood is screened in the U.K. and has been since October of last year and therefore we think it is safe. We have provided in a sense alternative sites for screening but not anonymous screening for patients in sexually transmitted clinics, we have also allowed people to be screened through general practitioners or primary care physicians.

A lot has been spoken about confidentiality and we put a lot of store in this. There is, in fact, an act of Parliament which says it is illegal to pass on information about a sexually acquired condition to any third party who is not involved in the clinical management of that patient. All of you who have worked in AIDS, I'm sure, have had very bad experiences in terms of confidentiality. We can all stand here and talk about how confidentiality is so important because we believe it is important and therefore it will be adhered to by everyone who works for us. But you only need two or three bad experiences to offset years of very hard work and for the public to believe that confidentiality is actually not working.

The fourth arm of control being developed in the U.K. is the development of guidelines for the protection of laboratory and clinical staff, similar guidance has been developed in the U.S.A. The final element of control, and the platform for all control is resources. In the U.K. in the last year just under four million pounds has been made available by the government for setting up counseling courses and providing money for some of the clinicians in London who have had to manage the majority of cases. Two million pounds was made available last year for changes within laboratories to make them safer and only 150 thousand pounds was put into the voluntary sector, particularly to the Terrence Higgins Trust.

We have not at the moment had problems in terms of hospital management of patients. There are three or four centers in London that manage most of the patients. But I do foresee that there will be considerable tension in the next year or two, as the number of cases within London increases. What happens is that not enough resources are put into a new problem. Even though I am a great advocate of the health service, one of the problems with it is that it finds it difficult to respond to a new crisis, particularly an epidemic of an infectious disease. So new money is not easily made available.

So, within the NHS one is able to look after AIDS patients but at a cost to other patients. The waiting lists for other operations and other conditions in fact gets longer. That obviously creates considerable tension between those of us who are looking after AIDS patients and our colleagues in a teaching hospital who feel that it is more appropriate that they should be looking after their transplant cases and their hip surgery and AIDS patients shouldn't be, as they put it, silting up the wards.

The final aspect is community care of patients. I'm full of admiration for the Shanti Project. I think that in certain areas in the United Kingdom we will have to develop services along that model. One of the problems that we face at the moment is, particularly in London, is that the National Health Service does not provide enough places for the chronically sick and dying.

Within the community there is the facility for patients to be managed by privacy call practitioners who have support staff such as district nurses who will go and nurse patients at home; a home help service, people who will go and clean and take food in to patients. All of these things will help people remain at home for as long as possible. All of those exist through the framework of the whole service. But I would not pretend that it works without problems. We've had considerable problems because of the anxiety, the hysteria, the fear of both medical and ancillary staff in the community who have been frightened to deal with AIDS patients. This is obviously changing.

**Sheldon Landesman, M.D.** (Associate Professor of Medicine, Director, AIDS Study Group, State Unversity of New York, Downstate Medical Center)

What I'd like to do with the time I have is to talk about the situation in New York City, how it is unique and different and uncomfortably bad in terms of the AIDS epidemic. I also want to talk a bit about policy debates that go on around dealing with the epidemic, focusing perhaps on New York City but realizing that these are things that can be generalized out to the entire debate on this epidemic well beyond the borders of the city.

New York City has had in excess of 6,000 cases of AIDS since this epidemic has started. Recent reports document approximately 220 to 250 new cases of AIDS reported to the City Department of Health each month. This probably represents an overall underestimate. There are an additional 20 to 25 percent of cases which are probably not reported to the Department of Health (DOH), in part because the Department of Health counts as AIDS cases only those that meet the CDC definition. Increasingly in New York City, particularly in public hospitals that are overburdened with these cases persons come in with bilateral diffuse infiltrates, are members of a risk group and get treated with TMX-Sulfa. They're put down within the local hospital statistics as PCP but in fact, are not counted by the city or the state or federal government as an AIDS case because they have not been histologically confirmed.

The same thing happens with toxoplasmosis. We see an increasing number of these cases in our hospital as well as in other hospitals in the city.

New York City, in terms of numbers, faces close to 300 new cases every month. To put that in some sort of perspective, that really is the equivalent to ten new patients every day of the week walking into hospitals here in the city and being diagnosed as having AIDS. It is an enormous problem.

Underlying the problem of the AIDS cases is the number of infected people here in the city. There are estimates from the Department of Health, and they appear to be conservative estimates, of 450,000 plus people who are infected with HIV here in the city. These are estimates because we haven't surveyed the entire city population. If the number 450,000 is correct, or close to correct, you're talking about five percent of the city population.

The case mix in New York City is different from what is reported nationally and has its own special flavor. Approximately 55 percent of the cases here in the city are in gay men, nearly 30 percent of the cases in the city are in IV drug users. Even though women compose a distinct minority of the cases of AIDS here in the city, it is of interest, if not of critical importance, to note that 20 percent of the women who have AIDS here in the city have been classified as sexual partners of risk group men. That number alone, I think, should put to rest the concept that this is a gay disease or a disease that is transmitted by anal-genital intercourse exclusively, or that anal, genital intercourse is dangerous whereas vaginal intercourse with an infected individual is safe.

An additional five percent of patients here in the city are listed as others or classified as unknowns. A significant proportion of that five percent are persons who have acquired the disease through heterosexual contact with a person that they did not know at that time was infected with the virus, and perhaps even the source of the infection did not know themselves that they were infected with the virus.

The impact of this epidemic on the hospitals here in New York City and on health care is, as you can imagine, immense. At our own hospital, we average between 20 and 30 patients on the in-house service of the hospital with approximately 180 to 200 total medical beds. Our house staff, to say the least, are discouraged.

An additional burden that we face here, which is one that is uncommonly faced elsewhere is the issue of pediatric AIDS. In our own hospital, we have anywhere from four to seven cases of pediatric AIDS on the ward at any one time. The pediatric service is much smaller than the medical service. The burdens that these babies put on the medical and nursing staff, to say nothing of the social service system here, are extraordinary. Compounding that problem are the large number of seropositive women of child-bearing age who bear children. In our ongoing study of pregnant methadone addicts, between 50 and 60 percent are seropositive. Most of these women have gone on to deliver their babies. We are in the process of evaluating what percentage of infected pregnant women give birth to infected infants.

It is important in that context to note that all seropositive pregnant women will give birth to an infant that is also seropositive. But the seropositivity is due to maternal antibody. You cannot in fact determine, given the present technology, whether an infant born of a seropositive mother is, in fact, infected until you wait anywhere from six months to a year and repeatedly test the child serologically, or unless the child develops symptomatic illness before that time.

There is a unique problem that we face. Often many of the children are taken away from their mothers because of continued drug use or poor care of the baby. You then face the issue of what to tell or who should tell the foster mother who cares for the baby what the status of the baby is when in fact we don't know.

Issues of confidentiality and what is appropriate then come to the fore, and those are some of the most difficult issues that we have had to deal with. The ones in the city at the present time are still unresolved ethical and moral questions.

Given the intensity of the problem that exists here in the city, it is not surprising that the debate here has been equally intense. Hopefully, everybody is well-meaning in their disagreement. Unfortunately part of the debate as it is carried out in the public sphere goes on with a lack of a certain element of scientific reality and goes on in a manner which only increases the problems. I'd like to give you some examples of them and try to suggest a mode to get out of this problem such that it could be useful to others in the future.

I think that one of the issues that serves as an example is the issue of heterosexual spread of this virus. There is no doubt in my mind nor in the mind of most other students of the disease that this is a sexually transmitted disease. HIV virus goes from man to man, man to women and perhaps, less efficiently from woman to man, but clearly is a sexually transmitted disease. I know of no sexually transmitted disease that goes unidirectionally and of no sexually transmitted disease that only goes with one type of intercourse. To hold it as anything other than a sexually transmitted disease or as transmitted through anal intercourse is to deny a certain reality that we will have to face because the disease itself won't listen to anything but its own biological imperatives.

Unfortunately, much of the debate on this disease in terms of its sexual transmission has centered around the concept of anal-genital sex being a dangerous activity. The implication being that vaginal intercourse is not dangerous. Often times, on our hotline we have in our hospital, we get calls from suburban housewives in Suffolk or Nassau County, saying that she and her husband have had anal-genital intercourse and can she now get AIDS from him. We try to explain to her that the critical factor is not how she has intercourse but whether or not her partner is infected.

But more important than the factor of misinformation to the public, believing that one type of intercourse is safe and another type is not safe is the misimpression that this sort of logic or this sort of public information gives to the public. I think that it is important to stress that when you classify one type of sexual activity associated with gay men as being dangerous, what you in fact do perhaps is assuage some of the fear and anxiety of the general heterosexual public which is probably one of the reasons it is done, although I don't know for certain. At the same time you separate out and split off one of the communities. You make the suburban housewife in Nassau or in Queens or in Suffolk feel comfortable that it is THEM who have the problem and WE don't have to worry about it. If and when the problem comes to that suburban housewife's door the first thing she is going to do is to blame it on THEM because they are not seen as a part of the community. Such artificial separation splits the community at a time when the community more than ever should not be split.

A similar sort of process occurs when you have newspaper journalists asking governmental officials, "Can this disease or is this disease spreading to the rest of the general population?" You should realize that that question has a very sort of subtle implication in it. It implies, at least for New York City, that the 400,000 infected people aren't part of the general population. It again reinforces the "them versus us" scenario that people tend to have with this sort of epidemic. It again splits the community rather than tending to bring it together. The sad thing is that sometimes the answer to that question is "No, it's not spreading to the general population, to the heterosexual population, it's just them."

Scientifically it is clear that spread into the heterosexual community is not a massive process. It will be slow, it'll be limited and it will probably be limited, to a great extent, at least in New York City, to the urban black and hispanic population, to the sexual partners of the drug users, and the sexual partners of the sexual partners. Nonetheless, there is a better answer to that question than the answer of plain simple no, which is perhaps scientifically incorrect, at least qualitatively, and somewhat misleading.

A better and more appropriate answer to that question is at the present time that this disease is largely confined to certain risk groups, but this is a disease that is sexually transmitted. The important point is that everybody in the general population and persons who are infected are part of the general population, should be aware of this and that this is a time of sexual selectivity and one has to be cautious, at least knowledgeable in selecting one's partners.

In the manner of public education, these sorts of answers are infinitely more useful in terms of preparing the public to deal with the disease and preparing the public for a willingness to support funding for the disease and to support measures needed to control the disease. It would also be useful in getting the risk groups affected and infected with this virus to, in fact, support public measures, which in a more hostile time may be looked upon as a curtailment of their civil liberties.

Another example of the issue of dealing with this disease, perhaps on the other side is the issue of HIV testing. My own personal belief is that testing is critical and important in controlling this epidemic. If you start with the ethical principle that nobody would knowingly want to infect anybody else with a potentially lethal disease, the knowledge that they have that capability and their duty then to inform their partner of that, I see as an important modifying factor in people's individual behavior.

However, because the many risk groups infected with the virus have been greatly concerned about the misuse of the test, they have somehow managed to convince other public officials to do what I call test bashing, which is to use spurious technological scientific arguments to deny the validity of this test. I won't go into all of the details of it now except to say that this has become so prevalent that many people in the general community and many scientific people who are familiar with the field continue to believe that the issue of testing evolves around the technological aspects of the tests and what it means when in fact it doesn't at all.

What can we do about taking these problems and trying to stop the epidemic, protecting civil liberties and protecting public health. We must, I believe, develop a new type of dialogue.

Solving the AIDS problem is not the issue of private civil rights versus the public good, not the issue of the individual versus society and not the issue of the minority versus the majority, which is the way it is seen by everybody. I would suggest a different way of seeing it. You can see it as everybody being part of a single societal community where everybody does something for the benefit of the community as a whole, starting out with the thesis that we are all in this together, rather than being separate.

This view of it leads to several different types of actions. For example, on the issue of testing in conjunction with counseling, and if behavior modification is all that we have at the present time and if behavior modification is dependent upon counseling and testing then the overriding public health goal would be to encourage people to be tested. However, we know that people won't be tested if they think that there is societal damage associated with testing, in terms of discrimination, loss of insurance, loss of job. So if we start with the model I have suggested, that we are all in this together and we have to do things for the communal good, we can then say two things. We can say that society should do everything it can to make sure it protects everybody that voluntarily comes forth to be tested in terms of health care, insurance and employment, while at the same time persons who are infected should then come forth to be tested in an environment where they are protected and they can protect their fellow citizens.

If we include everybody in our societal framework, if we protect those whose cooperation we need in order for them to protect others, then maybe we can accomplish more in this epidemic than we have accomplished to date.

Eric Sandstrom, M.D., Ph.D. (Associate Professor, Department of Dermatology-Venereology, Karolinska Institute, Stockholm, Sweden, Secretary, Swedish Government Delegation on AIDS)

It has been stated in the introduction that HIV infection knows no geographical boundaries. This conference bears witness to this with representatives from many different states around the world and in the United States. To put Sweden, a country of eight million people, in the perspective of the United States, we would rank as the 27th state together with Hawaii with regard to AIDS incidence. In this talk I will briefly describe the kind of legislation that has been implemented in Sweden and the effects that we are currently witnessing.

AIDS in Sweden is principally a problem of the major cities with few cases reported in other parts of the country. Ninety percent of the cases have been found in the gay community. Twenty percent of those classified as homosexual men also report heterosexual activity. Two cases are reported that are probably due to heterosexual spread.

Prior to the clinical reporting that I will describe there was a voluntary laboratory reporting of test results to the National Bacteriological Laboratory. In most of the reported cases risk group, age, and sex were stated. This reporting, however, was carried out under a number of different codes, so that double reporting can not be excluded. The statistics continue to be accumulated and serve as a quality control to the public health reporting.

In the course of the collection of these statistics it was discovered that HIV infection was spreading among IV drug users in Stockholm. This sparked a public debate over the regulations in Sweden. The debate focused on the fact that some of the infected people were found to be heroin addicts and support themselves as prostitutes. The proponents of a law regulating HIV infections claim that society had a right to intervene in the freedom of the individual to curb disease spread. Others claimed it was counterproductive since infected people would avoid seeking medical care for their problems and thus a net increase in spread would result. Gay activists and others voiced their fears of registration, discrimination and the possibility of involuntary confinement.

The Swedish law on communicable diseases has two sections. One section deals with a broad scope of communicable diseases and a smaller section with venereal diseases in particular. Among the differences is that confidentiality is taken into account in the venereal disease section. However, in the latter section there was a clause stating a two-year jail sentence if a patient had sex while infected and untreated. It was elected to include HIV infections among the venereal diseases, but at the same time removing the possibility to imprison patients that did not conform. Thus both proponents and opponents to the law tended to view the law as a means to reach the few that continue to spread disease in spite of society's efforts to persuade them not to. The provision that remain under the law was to confine such a person to a hospital until he or she is non-infectious.

The change in the law was enacted the first of November 1985. It stated that anyone that suspects that he or she could have been infected with HIV should seek medical attention for testing. The "suspicion" is defined as someone that has had sex with someone known to be HIV positive or have shared syringes or needles with somebody known to be infected by HIV. A person named as a contact to somebody that is HIV seropositive can also be required to undergo HIV testing.

The law did, however, have an additional number of effects. The responsibilities of the physicians were firmly regulated. For instance, a physician can not test anybody without informed consent, except if that person is referred as a contact. Furthermore the physician has to assume full responsibility for the clinical handling of the patients should the test prove to be positive. If the physician is not prepared to take this responsibility, the patient should be referred to a center that can do so. The physician has to offer testing under code. Once a positive test result is obtained the doctor is responsible for giving full information on all aspects of HIV infection including what precautions should be taken to avoid spreading the virus further. Regular follow-ups have to be offered in addition to psychosocial support for the patients and those that are next of kin to the patients. Since HIV is regulated as a venereal disease these services are offered free of charge. The physician is required to perform contact tracing, but not to report his findings to the public health officer if he is taking responsibility for the epidemiological work-up. In practice the epidemiological work-up consists of a thorough information on how the infection was introduced into the country and a thorough discussion of the particular patient's life style during that period. Thus partners present themselves at the request of the patient. Doctors have elected to report very few contacts further to the public health officer. Positive test results, risk group, age and sex, is reported under code to the public health officer who compiles the data and sends them further to the National Bacterological Laboratory for further analysis.

There has been a marked improvement of the performance of many authorities as a result of the law. A government level delegation has been formed with political representatives, the representatives of the major authorities. Thus the existence of the law and the delegation clearly spells out to all concerned in governmental and administrative work that HIV infection is a national priority. The situation that prompted the enactment of the law, has been tested in court you can forcefully confine a patient who continues to spread disease. The law states the clinician should report such a patient to the public health officer who in turn should test the case in court. If the court agrees, the individual can be confined in a infectious disease hospital. A heroin addict maintained that he behaved the way he did so that disease could be spread. He was subsequently confined with two guardians in an infectious disease hospital, but released after three weeks into an open program for his drug addiction. It was concluded that the present law is not suited to forcefully deal with HIV infection, particularly not in drug addicts. However, that part of the law has hardly ever been used before in the handling of venereal diseases. The strength of the law has always been the regulation of epidemiological work and patient care.

The evaluation of the ultimate acceptance of the law by high risk groups is however complicated by the effect of other laws. As of January 1, 1986, another law came into effect that among other things stated that all medical records should carry the full identification on the concerned individual. This was in conflict with practice of anonymous HIV screening. It again sparked the debate over possibilities of registration and discrimination. In May, this law was changed so that testing could be carried out anonymously while medical treatments should be done with a full identification to ensure the reliability of medical records.

This fall, changes in laws will take place that enable the public health officer to obtain further information on patients that are supposed to continue to spread disease. Although there is political unity as to the safeguards with respect to the personal integrity the political goals are again questioned in the public debate.

The authorities and clinicians have conformed to the law and have now caught up with a number of cases identified through the laboratory reports. There was a sharp decline in attendance for HIV screening particularly among gay men during the winter 1985/1986. This was particularly true for men that turned out to test positive. The decline was in the order of 30 percent with most attendees requiring full anonymity. Numbers are slowly beginning to rise again. About half of those reported consist of gay men (of whom 25 percent also have had sex with women). The most rapid increase of reported cases has been in IV drug users. This is a problem currently confined to the major metropolitan area of Stockholm. Among those using amphetamines intravenously (about 7,500) about 5 percent are currently judged to be positive.

There are clear indications that we see heterosexual spread of HIV infection in Sweden. This means that in our strategical considerations we, from the outset have to design information and education especially for the younger heterosexual population.

The information effort in Sweden started as in many other places in the gay community as a result of the efforts of concerned gay individuals and the national gay organization. A county supported gay health screening project was initiated in Stockholm before the first case of AIDS was diagnosed in Sweden. National authorities were however slower to respond to the epidemic. Over the last year there has been a surge of interest with an increased amount of media coverage and activities from authorities on all levels. Drug abuse programs have been beefed up with the ultimate goal to reach every IV drug user in the country (estimated to number about 20,000). A national strategy has been funded with the equivalent of about $40 million over two years focusing on information, psychosocial support and IV drug abuse programs.

Basic to our epidemiological efforts is HIV antibody testing. We have of course had the same controversy over the appropriate use of the HIV tests as other societies. Opponents claim there is an inherent risk of registration and subsequent discrimination. Potentially infected individuals might not seek medical attention and thus increase rather than decrease the spread of HIV. Furthermore, all members of risk groups should modify their behavior in order to decrease the risk of spreading HIV regardless if they test positive at any one time or not.

However, if HIV seropositivity is to be used as a means to follow the spread of the epidemic, representative large scale testing is mandatory while maintaining a high quality of the collected data. Thus there should be no fear of registration. There should be a benefit to the person that is being tested. For those negative (which is currently 96 percent of gay men) there is a relief from anxiety and a provision of enough information on how to stay uninfected. For those testing positive there should be high quality psychosocial and medical care. The collected statistics should be made public and discussed to strengthen the understanding that it is important to follow the actual spread of infection rather than settling for clinical outcomes that reflect what happened several years ago.

Furthermore the change of behavior is difficult, but most people that learn they are infected are eager to take the difficult steps necessary to protect their loved ones. The people seen in the testing situation are very receptive to information. These individuals will turn out to be the best educators in the very communities that we wish to reach. We can in this situation identify hidden psychosocial needs and try to meet them. In our efforts we try to provide hepatitis-B vaccine to those who have not had hepatitis-B in an effort to eradicate this disease as a bonus.

It is worth stressing that this kind of program is not possible if you are not ready to provide good psychosocial support from voluntary networks and professionals. As in other places gay men have made great contributions.

We are all overwhelmed by the magnitude of the problem in high prevalence areas such as New York, San Francisco and Los Angeles. The policies that are by necessity adopted in these areas may not be suitable for areas with lower prevalence of HIV infection but might be able to afford other strategies and in the process, learn from each other.

Session D:  Education and Communication:  Enhancing Public
Understanding and Fostering Disease Prevention

## Participants

### Speakers

Nathan Fain
Freelance Journalist

Robert Bazell
Science Correspondent, NBC News

### Panelists

Virginia Apuzzo
Deputy Executive Director, New York State Consumer Protection
Board

Jim Bunn
Reporter, KPIX-TV, San Francisco

Michael Callen
New York State AIDS Advisory Council, Member, People with AIDS
Coalition

Andrew Veitch
Medical Correspondent, The Guardian, London, England

Tony Whitehead
Chairperson, Terrence Higgins Trust, London, England

EDUCATION AND COMMUNICATION:  ENHANCING PUBLIC UNDERSTANDING AND

FOSTERING DISEASE PREVENTION

Virginia Apuzzo[1],
Nathan Fain[2], and
Robert Bazell[3]

INTRODUCTION


Ms. Apuzzo

I'd like to take a few moments to describe to you how we will
proceed in this session.  We will have two presentations, one by
Mr. Fain and one by Mr. Bazell, and then we will have an
opportunity for each of the four panelists to provide you with a
thumbnail sketch of their perspectives as they interact with each
other and specifically with the two speakers.  The emphasis during
this session will be the extent to which the media, electronic and
print, has enhanced public understanding and fostered disease
prevention.  As moderator, I must confess that I found it difficult
to be moderate, on this point.  I've found it difficult to be
moderate because, as Executive Director of the National Gay Task
Force, during the first three or four years of the AIDS epidemic I
have experienced first hand a litany of things that have given me
reason to question the media.  Indeed there were incidents in the
initial months and some would say years of the AIDS epidemic, in
which our very grip on reality was questioned.

One example that comes to mind is the fact that after the New
York Times discovered AIDS in its news pages, declared the
existence of an epidemic, tallied deaths here in New York and then
San Francisco, we couldn't find any indication of it in the
obituary pages.  We had the establishment of institutions in the
gay community that were funded and resourced by members of the
community, we put on events, such as filling Madison Square Garden
in a major fund raising event and there was no trace in the media
of what was happening within the most affected community.

While gay newspapers carried ground breaking news on the
existence of the disease, there are hundreds of thousands of gay

[1]  Deputy Executive Director, New York State Consumer Protection
Board  [2]  Freelance Journalist  [3]  Science Correspondent, NBC
News

men who for reasons that are personal to them have no access to these gay newspapers.

They thus remained ignorant and as such vulnerable. The list can go on and on. We've seen hysteria from the media. We've seen words like quarantine. We've seen Mr. Buckley talk about tattooing at least twice in the last several months. We've been dazzled by complexity and we have been stunned by simplicity.


DISCUSSION


### Mr. Fain

I'm told we're here today to talk about what part the media plays, has played, ought to play, in the enhancement of public understanding and the fostering of disease prevention. In other words, how do we get radio, television and the press to alert the public to a health threat, in the case of AIDS a very complicated and conditional threat, without causing more harm than good? By the very language I have just used to describe the problem, I may have offended several of you, I hope not the majority. But I would like to apply my own experience writing about AIDS directly to the heart of this problem.

I have tried for several years to get the story out as cleanly as I found it and my experience has taught me that the problem is inherently philosophical, clouded by such difficult matters as the decline of the clear use of language, the corruption of trust and authority, the blurring of useful distinctions. In war and in advertising, we call this use of language propaganda, that is, information that is no longer neutral but has been conscripted into serving a cause. Whatever you might think AIDS is, you might consider also that it is a frontal attack on the machinery of language and therefore on the very underpinnings of civilized order itself.

A quick word about my so-called experience. I was brought up, educated and trained as a journalist. I have worked in daily, weekly and monthly print in radio and television. I haven't seen it all but I've seen some of it. When the first reports of the epidemic appeared on July 3, 1981, I sensed that a big story was unfolding, so that my concern for my own safety was from the beginning offset by a kind of awe that any journalist feels when he knows he has walked into the largest event he will ever witness.

War correspondents know this feeling very well. That AIDS was to become the Vietnam of an emerging self-identified sector of the international male population seemed possible but remote back in 1981.

Nevertheless, by early 1982 a number of friends and I recognized that a situation of the first gravity was upon us. And for reasons that I may not go into now, we knew that almost alone, we were going to have to do something about it. We started a foundation, named it Gay Men's Health Crisis and began as best we could planning a number of defenses against this bizarre disease.

Our first line of defense was knowledge. My good friend Dr. Lawrence Mass owns the singular honor of being the first person to write in depth about this epidemic in an impressive series of pieces in the city's gay newspaper, The Native. Shortly after I began a similar service for a national publication called the Advocate. He and I together took it upon ourselves to investigate the situation and report to our own people as it were, to gay men and women, just what we could find out about the disease.

We had begun GMHC, in fact, on the principal that no one physician had a hammerlock on AIDS as one or two of them tried to tell us they did have.

Larry and I made a lot of mistakes. Looking back, I think the biggest mistake we made was that we both exhausted ourselves trying to get the facts straight. He even more than I, lost a lot of sleep worrying over the smallest details. We got to know Jim Curran at the CDC awfully well, not to mention dozens of other physicians all over the country and pretty soon the Western World.

We sifted through some of the zaniest opinions we had ever encountered and tried to hit a resonant middle note, a consensus, a sophisticated and reasoned assessment of what was after all, a scenario that approached, as Michael Gottlieb at UCLA told me at the time, science fiction.

Well, I think Larry and I more or less blew it. We don't congratulate ourselves, not only did we recognize that we were alone, that very few people really were interested in the facts. We also came to recognize that the news we had brought, and all the careful ways we were delivering it to other gay men, was the worst possible story we could have given them. It detonated their deepest fears. It was like reporting a new and embarrassing genetic defect linked by race. We put a little too much faith in the strength of heart of people who are finally people. We believed the fallacy that being gay meant being better, stronger, smarter. It is an unfair and inhumane assumption, a trap into which many oppressed people fall.

We tried, I think, to defend ourselves from having to deal with this extra dimension by clinging with religious zeal to the facts, to what you might call objective reality and most fatally, we insisted as founders and board members, that GMHC proceed at a sober and steady pace to protect its credibility and to avoid being dismissed by our readers as madly and unduly alarmist. Above all, we felt GMHC should provide reliable information and then stand discreetly aside to allow people to make whatever changes in their lives they saw fit. And therefore, accept responsibility for those changes.

We were not about to be drawn into a parent/child relationship acting in loco parentis. To do so, we felt, was to seal indictments from our worst enemies, inside and outside medicine, people who said we are immature and compulsive, perhaps subhuman, incapable of discharging the duties of full American citizenship. Of course, the ultimate question, then as now, was how alarmist is unduly alarmist? I would guess that we still don't have many answers, although the situation has aged enough to have lost some of its early centrifugal force.

I think the argument will never be settled, not in my lifetime anyway.  As alarming as AIDS is, it's not the first or even the greatest danger that faces the entire world.  And no matter how much a person reads, hears, or sees about AIDS, his or her feelings about it seemed governed more by direct contact with the disease.

It is not an intellectual process, it is glandular and immediate.  No words can contain it.  The barrier that Dr. Mass and I faced in the early days was the very human desire to avoid bad news.  One part of our gay leadership seemed prepared to defend sexual freedom to the limit, that limit being defined as the risk of death itself; the other part was prepared to defend gay political integrity and indeed life itself by advocating total sexual shutdown.  And this long before we knew much at all about the natural history of AIDS.

Nothing we wrote persuaded either side toward moderation.  As you know, what happened from the fall of 1981 until the spring of 1983 was that very little appeared outside the gay press about AIDS because the problem seemed to be confined pretty much to us.  People tend not to worry about threats to others.  If the Chernobyl fallout had drifted only over Soviet real estate, I doubt that world concern would have reached the proportions it has.  The Europeans certainly got more excited than we did.

Owing to the main route of entry the AIDS virus took in North America, to the central role in transmission played by the blood stream, AIDS was considered unworthy of concern paid to, say, the great epidemics of history that have killed tens of millions of people via airborne antigens.  Even in our own century, an onslaught of post-World War I pneumonia left twenty million dead.  Now that is an epidemic, or so any overtaxed news editor will tell you.

This general judgment remains today the most alienating, the simple calculation of numbers likely to be affected by this disease.  Debate continues, as you know, over just how endangered is the "general population", to use the deathless phrase of the late Secretary of Health and Human Services, Margaret Heckler.

Because AIDS at first seemed so selective, the people it mostly selected were immediately suspicious of a plot.  Many are to this day, I regret to point out, fearing the attitude of the mainstream press about whether these men deserve to die.  This attitude was not very carefully disguised.  One of the more overt expressions of that joy at the pain of others, the German word is Schadenfreude, appeared in 1983 in the Sunday magazine of the New York Times, wherein a writer referred to infant cases of AIDS as "innocent victims".  Adults with AIDS must have earned their misery, the Times implied.

A few months after that, the same newspaper put an extremely misleading headline on an AP dispatch about a medical journal paper that discussed the possibility that "major household contact" might spread the AIDS germ.  I won't mention the journal or the author of the paper but I'm sure you all know to whom I refer.  This collusion of clear sense led to a summer of media hysteria and public excitement.

The nation not only woke up but proceeded immediately to a full psychotic break. Suddenly the disease thought to have some exclusive preference for homosexual men and needle users was stalking middle America. As a cover line on Life magazine declared, nobody was safe. As you know, the craziness persisted as late as last September, when parents all over America kept their children from schools on grounds of deep mistrust of statements from public health officers. What it came down to was, for the parents, that no medical authority could honestly say, that their children were absolutely, completely safe. I wrote several pieces myself about this issue and I tried very hard to arrive at language that sounded like one hundred percent certainty, even though I could not of course find one physician who could give me such a quote. What I had to stitch together was a crude line of logic that tried to overwhelm the skeptic, and the obtainable facts of the matter were and still are contradictory in the extreme.

Probabilities are one thing that people, particularly parents, want to be sure of. We cannot, of course, be absolutely sure of anything but death, and Plato long ago shot a hole in even that certainty by pointing out that it was the highest arrogance of man to be afraid of death, since we could not know what lay on the other side of it. Maybe death is terrific, Plato said, we simply don't know. But the certainty people want, certainty that the sun will rise in the east tomorrow is not to be had in much of science, especially not in medical science. The component facts about AIDS are, to this day, so prismatic and controversial that you can project just about any agenda you have onto them and force it through the prism.

The point is obvious, that combining sex and death gives you a story unlike any other, unlike even nuclear annihilation, which we do not expect as a consequence of sexual pleasure.

I propose that it is therefore virtually impossible to strike the right tone in print about AIDS, not too hysterical, not too relaxed, not too much nor too little. The public in general and even in particular is far too alienated from their deepest fears to comprehend the factual direct message without rebelling.

Inviting people to trust the information you are giving them, then hoping they will act responsibly on that information, was and remains extremely tricky. A major point of argument, for example, involves whether such a thing as so-called safe sex or more technically infection-free sex, is even possible. A number of gay men say it is, but another number say it is not. Many experts disagree and arguments over how frankly this kind of sex should be talked about has delayed for nearly a year badly needed federal funding to programs planned by GMHC and similar foundations. A delay Paul Volberding of San Francisco rightly terms a scandal.

You might imagine also gay men are inclined to trust their own press, more than they trust the other general press. This is not always so; information about AIDS is believed by any gay man in direct proportion to its distance from a statistical authority, especially in New York. That you might anticipate this phenomenon among people who are not highly educated whether they are gay or not is beside the point. You would expect it among, say, drug addicts who are almost by definition focused on one thing, drugs.

You would rightly expect it among Haitian immigrants, people who have fled such a wretched existence that most of us cannot imagine how wretched it is, because the existence they enjoy in our country looks pretty wretched to us and yet we know they risk their lives to obtain it. We might even have expected such a wall of alienation from an entire government, such as the Soviet Union and virtually all those on the African continent have elected to take about AIDS.

Only last night, as I was going over this address, I heard a television report, that Uganda has now revealed for the first time that it does indeed have cases of AIDS, 500 of them, in fact. We can agree from a smug distance from our perch over here that it is shocking how little cooperation science is getting from these governments. Denial on a grand scale, I admit, yet hardly a new phenomenon. But I will tell you how it came to pass that I was the shocked, seasoned reporter that I am supposed to be. My own shock came when I began to realize how deeply suspicious were many of my fellow gay men who were in fact far more educated than I. I'm speaking of people at the doctorate level, products of medical schools and the highest research institutions, the best universities, the actual five-star longheads in virology, epidemiology, and so on. People who had fought hard to succeed in a world rather hostile to manifestations of their private tastes in affection. This exists not only in America but in Europe and Australia, South Africa. Their distrust, their suspicion of the academy and their governments approaches total meltdown, I think. By definition, these people work in the establishment but by temperament, when their own lives are threatened and the lives of those they love, they are as alienated from authority as any dissident Soviet physicist.

All their massive intellectual machinery subverts them at the critical point when they are confronted with rhetorical evidence that suggests they may die a horrible death. Because their life-long effort to erect the machinery was in part an act of defiance against a society that they knew would be delighted if they simply vanished from sight. I sometimes think that the gay physician, the gay scientist is the ultimate existentialist and not the late criminal poet, Jean Genet, who by comparison was only going through the motions.

Another simpler way to say what I mean is to cast a glance at a contemporary of Genet's, the novelist William Burroughs, a failed physician, long user of opiates, classically suspicious of all voices of government and authority and even of civilization itself. Burroughs' character is a prophetic analogy between the invasion of the body by a virus and the invasion of the soul by propaganda and hate.

I quote a chilling sentence from his novel Ah Pook Is Here, published in the fatal year 1979. "A virus is a living picture that makes itself out of you." Most of his work is about this analogy between propaganda and infection. In the minds of some intellectual gay men, it is accepted that Burroughs predicted the epidemic as a grand paranoid nightmare. A deliberate act. Whether this idea can be proved or not doesn't matter to those who believe it. To them, faith is beyond fact, and superior to it. We are now outside the realm of philosophy, itself a pursuit rendered useless to us by its arcane progressions and systems theory.

It would seem as though we are no better now than savages when a big crisis erupts; all our fancy structures don't work the way they were designed to work. The proof of that statement is that we are so reluctant in the face of failure to admit failure. We are reluctant to recognize what my colleague Ginny Apuzzo calls the primitive heart, which I think she understands far better than I. You are more fortunate than you know to have her here today to moderate the discussion that follows me, because she knows better than any of us what I am talking about.

It seems to me that the crisis AIDS presents is very much like the crisis that reckless handling of nuclear energy presents. They are both in a sense disorders of civilization, symptoms that indicate something is out of whack. I don't mean to suggest that both disasters had to happen, sooner or later. My point is really in the opposite direction, that the world's larger mechanisms, its capacity to deal with big time danger by communicating reliable warnings, obviously does not work very well.

Some components of it work very well indeed, the more technical the more impressive, but these technical stunts seem to throw into even sharper relief the fissures and craters in our political systems. The more exact, the more specific reporting on AIDS has become, I have noticed, the more profoundly alienated those immediately involved have become. It is as though what we call understanding is rendered useless. I would go further and propose that the error here lies in the way the media has used language to warn. Usually language is limited by the haste imposed by the very technical nature of the industry. I won't belabor the point, but you know what the term hit-and-run journalism means, yet the twentieth century can be regarded as an encyclopedia of the unheeded warning or else the tardy warning.

Most of these warnings were clear, simple, and direct. They were not issued in the present overstimulated atmosphere. It has fallen to me to have become one of the warners myself, enjoying pretty fast company with those who warned of Hitler, of Pearl Harbor, of all our demons. What we share, these people and I, is the experience of having tried to tell the truth and then watched as something other than the truth, maybe higher, I admit, was allowed to prevail, to shape policy.

I doubt that it comforts any of these early warners. It certainly doesn't comfort me to know that they saw the disaster coming sooner than most. In point of fact, I can describe the feeling as much like watching an automobile skid across a slick highway toward its certain target. Joseph Heller gave a new word to our language, a word that describes neatly the little problem I have been talking about, and I quote, "There was only one catch, and that was Catch-22, which specified that a concern for one's safety in the face of dangers that were real and immediate, was the process of a rational mind." If you go back through all that has been broadcast and printed in this country about AIDS, much of it will seem rational, some of it not. But whatever your opinion, only a little of it is total gibberish. It took the checkout tabloid press a long time to dive into AIDS, for example, as late as the Rock Hudson story, because the thing was just too outlandish even for them. They couldn't get a handle on it beyond the occasional item like my favorite, about a retired San Diego pathologist and amateur archaeologist featured in one of these tabloids. In his opinion, a viral curse had been placed in the sarcophagus of King Tut, the bug having got out as planned during the King's recent tour of America. Why here? Why now? The pathologist somehow had inside information that the priests of Egypt foresaw a period of licentious libertarianism and had prepared just the medicine for its cure.

This you expect, but how prepared were we to accept the suggestion from our resident national keeper of high rationality, William Buckley himself, that all seropositive citizens be tattooed? We face an utilitarian imperative, wrote Buckley in the Times last March. Roll that phrase over your tongue and savor its subtle, may I add deadly, taste. It is easy to make fun of Buckley and many have, but I won't; I don't think I am any better than he is, I also faced a utilitarian imperative although in my own defense I didn't reach for quite such a symbiotic over-simplification as the tattoo. What I did reach for was my journeyman training, my inadequate education at the hands of the school of journalism of the University of Texas. It was okay, but it wasn't enough. It was in fact boring. It was too balanced, too cool, too professional.

Others took another route in the gay press and outside it. Some of the most overwrought heliotrope prose has defaced perfectly good newsprint in the cause of AIDS. A recent national magazine award was bestowed on a major article that was loaded with factual mistakes but had a second act curtain that must have reached the judges in their entrails. A certain play has been bought as we say for the movies, a play that will probably advance sympathy for disease victims as no printed word can. But every word of the play is a lie, to borrow from Mary McCarthy, including "and" and "the". Common wisdom says the time must pass for even superficial journalism much less real literature to take the measure of AIDS correctly. It's a poor excuse but I believe here is the real problem with writing about AIDS. We must cover its news, but we do so heartlessly, recognizing how futile the exercise really is. Such a confusing swarm of information is bound to fail to transmit, to connect because the emotional factor is too great.

As with all that has been written about the threat of nuclear war, we think we have made the point, warned the public, alerted our government, done our jobs, we journalists surely deserve a pat on the head. I know quite a few of my colleagues who regard themselves as veritable heroes for their work in AIDS. They may yet prove to be so. In the meantime I remain skeptical if not cynical, convinced only that we are witnessing one more blind spasm of history. Technically, we are right on top of the story, morally we are not. No news there of course, but I wonder these days how much it will take to advance our understanding of life so that our future warnings may be confined to natural disasters that are not amplified by human blindness. Thank you.


## Mr. Bazell

I have the distinction of being the only representative here of the national American general media. I accept the challenge, if it is that; I certainly don't view myself as any sort of hero and I'm very happy to have been invited.

I do want to point out, however, that I don't work for the New York Times, I don't work for ABC or CBS, I only work for NBC and what I'm going to do is present six of my own pieces that all appeared on the NBC Nightly News in the last four years. My hope by doing this is to focus the discussion to some specifics because I would like to share with you the thoughts that I had in putting these pieces together and the difficulties that I encountered. I also welcome your criticisms of how this might have been done better at the time, and what's much more important, what can be done for the future.

Now you might say that it's both egotistical and stupid of me to sit here and show you six of my pieces but I know those who say that to be a television correspondent you have to be egotistical and stupid. I will proceed.

This first piece appeared on June 17, 1982. I too, like Nathan, had been interested in the AIDS epidemic since 1981 when I first heard about it.

I have a background of training in science and immunology and I found it fascinating for its public health implications as well as for its implications for basic science. However, I wasn't successful in convincing my producers to put a piece on until June 16, 1982, that was the date that the MMWR appeared with the cohort study showing that AIDS was transmitted by sexual activity and to my knowledge this is the first American network television presentation on AIDS.

TOM BROKAW: ...Today they released the results of a study which shows that the lifestyle of some male homosexuals has triggered an epidemic of a rare form of cancer. Robert Bazell now in Atlanta...

ROBERT BAZELL: Robert Campbell of San Francisco and Billy Rocker of New York both suffer from a serious newly discovered disease which affects mostly homosexual men but has also been found in heterosexual men and women. The condition severely weakens the body's ability to fight disease. Many victims get a rare form of cancer called Kaposi's Sarcoma, others get an infection known as pneumocystis pneumonia. Researchers know of 413 people who have contracted the condition in the past year. One third have died and none have been cured.

ROBERT BAZELL: Investigators have examined the habits of homosexuals for clues.

INTERVIEWEE: I was in the fast lane at the time because of the way I lived my life and now I'm not.

ROBERT BAZELL: The best guess is that some infectious agent is causing it. Today researchers here at the National Centers for Disease Control said they had found several cases where people who have been sex partners both had the condition.

The scientists say this probably means they are dealing with some new deadly sexually transmitted disease. Investigators see this as a serious public health problem from an epidemic point of view, there have been more deaths from Kaposi's Sarcoma and pneumocystis pneumonia than have occurred with all the cases of Toxic Shock Syndrome and the Philadelphia outbreak of Legionnaire's disease combined.

Researchers are now studying blood and other samples from the victims trying to learn what is causing the disease. So far they have no luck. Robert Bazell, NBC News, Atlanta.

Okay, so now we are going to jump ahead to the next year. We are going to go to June 21, 1983. During this year, my colleagues did several cases, several pieces, emphasizing different research findings, the geometric increase of the disease and that sort of thing. I wish I had time to show you more but looking back on that first piece, I think the best thing in it was what Jim Curran said comparing it to Legionnaire's disease and Toxic Shock because as much difficulty as we had getting that story, both Legionnaire's disease and Toxic Shock had received an enormous amount of publicity at the time that they occurred.

So drawing that comparison from my standpoint was very important. In the meantime there were major developments in the four H's, the homosexuals, the heroin users, the hemophiliacs and the Haitians? And with amazingly little difficulty I took a camera crew and went to Haiti. It really wasn't that difficult, and the thing that was amazing to me was that I think I was the first reporter from the general press, either television or print, to go to Haiti to try to find out what was going on. It was not easy and we certainly got no cooperation there, but I did come up with this report which I would like to show you now.

ANCHORMAN: Federal health officials and a representative from the White House met today in Washington with representatives from six homosexuals' organizations to explore what the administration is doing about the disease called AIDS, Acquired Immune Deficiency Syndrome. The government today outlined a series of research projects underway to find a treatment towards a cure for the deadly disease.

Most often AIDS strikes homosexual men, drug addicts, and surprisingly Haitians. In the second of two reports science correspondent Robert Bazell looks at the mysterious Haitian connection.

ROBERT BAZELL: Haiti is the poorest country in the Western hemisphere. AIDS, the deadly new disease, is a growing problem here. More than 150 cases have been diagnosed. Most of the AIDS cases have been treated here at the University of Haiti Hospital in Port-au-Prince. The doctors who are treating the patients have been told by the government not to be interviewed on television.

Haitian doctors in the United States told us that many of the victims are from Caufo and the poverty suburb of Port-au-Prince. At night the district becomes, as one doctor put it, similar to the 42nd Street and Time Square area where males and females compete with each other for the business they need to survive.

Many tourist bars are full of prostitutes. In Chez Denise, we use the hidden camera and the microphone to speak to the

owners. He said Chez Denise caters soley to homosexuals,
mostly from the United States. Hundreds of local men and boys
and working prostitutes meet their foreign born customers at
Chez Denise. There is no way they can get a job and they get
paid for giving them a good deal. They'll do whatever you
want, for money.

AIDS first appeared among recent Haitian immigrants of the
United States. American doctors interviewing them concluded
they were neither homosexuals nor drug addicts. So the U.S.
government declared that Haitians for some unknown reason run a
risk of contracting AIDS. Haitian doctors say that the
interviews were not conducted properly.

SPEAKER: Most of those people may be illegal, they don't speak
English very well and homosexuality is not something that is
accepted in Haiti. It's a taboo and it's very hard for someone
to say I am gay and I have had sexual activities in the past.

ROBERT BAZELL: The Haitian doctors say interviews they have
done reveal that at least one fourth of the Haitian AIDS
victims worked as male prostitutes. So called folk doctors
like Dr. Napo whose offices are in a back alley of a
Port-au-Prince slum. This is thought to be another reason for
this threat of AIDS among the Haitians.

SPEAKER: Most cannot afford to see a trained physician.
Instead they take a number and pay two dollars to wait to see
the folk doctor. Dr. Napo told us he got his medical degree
through a correspondence course. He gives a quick examination
and then orders medication. Often his assistant injects it.
Once she is done she throws the needles and syringe into a bowl
of water so they can be used again on another patient. Haitian
physicians say that such use of dirty needles is common and may
be spreading AIDS among Haitians in the same way that dirty
needles spread the disease among American drug addicts.

SPEAKER: They know that there is no evidence for saying that
AIDS came from here in Haiti to the United States. In fact it
could just as well have gone the other way.

SPEAKER: But there is real fear. Many Americans have
cancelled their reservations at Haiti's luxury hotels. And
Haitians living in the United States say they are feared and
discriminated against because of AIDS.

SPEAKER: My mother lost a job in a factory because many people
see Haitians as people who have AIDS.

SPEAKER: He lost his job after working there for a year with
this couple. They decided that all Haitians had AIDS and they
let him go.

ROBERT BAZELL: The facts indicate AIDS is not a Haitian
disease. It is transmitted among Haitians just as it is in the
United States. Mostly by sexual contact and dirty needles.
Robert Bazell, NBC News, Port-au-Prince.

Just a quick comment on that piece before I go on. The biggest
problem that I had with that piece was something right in the
middle of it and this is in terms of any of you who are journalists

or any of you who are physicians that deal with television; it had nothing to do with Haiti. There was a middle picture of Dr. Rubenstein who is at Albert Einstein Medical College here in New York and some of his colleagues examining a Haitian patient and the patient had active pneumocystis and the hospital required that they be wearing masks at the time because of the pneumonia. I didn't know anything about that, I wasn't even thinking about it, but it turned out that the image of those people wearing masks and examining that AIDS patient persisted. Television doesn't convey facts very well but it sure conveys images very well, in an excellent way, and that was a big mistake. It wasn't just my mistake. To show doctors and nurses with masks around an AIDS patient at that point particularly, in 1983, was a big mistake.

The other comment that I would make quickly on that piece before we move on is, that the piece was essentially advocacy journalism on my part. There hadn't been much study of the Haitian issue and I think that there was something going on with the Haitians in the same way that there is something going on in Africa. The Haitians were getting a bad rap and I don't think the issue had been investigated clearly at that point, so I took a stand. I didn't take a position but I did take a stand that certainly offered a point of view.

We are going to move ahead a few years. We're skipping 1984, going ahead to what was one piece of a series about AIDS that I did over time, as often as I could, which wasn't as often as I wanted to.

What was important about this piece is that I had gone to San Francisco General Hospital and shot this piece. I was planning to take several days, as I usually would to put it together. In fact, that afternoon when Rock Hudson got sick his spokesman said he had AIDS or something like that and I had to throw it together in three hours, so it could run on the air that night because suddenly the producers for whom I work had an enormous interest in AIDS, much more than they had had before.

ROBERT BAZELL: This is the AIDS clinic at the San Francisco General Hospital. Here one can begin to understand the magnitude of the AIDS epidemic and the meaning of the growing numbers of new cases and deaths. Ron Carey learned that he had AIDS three and a half years ago. He is one of the longest surviving AIDS patients in the world. Most die between 6 months and two years after they are diagnosed. Ron Carey has seen a lot of people die.

RON CAREY: I have lost 74 close friends in the course of this disease. I've known a lot more than that over the last three years.

ROBERT BAZELL: The staff members all volunteer here for the jobs. Most days they handle them well, sometimes it gets tough.

SPEAKER: There was a time about a week ago, where in 20 days we had more than 20 deaths, every once in a while I feel like throwing up my hands and saying I am going to go to work in a clinic where I am working with mothers and babies, people who are well. Because I want to see people who get better. And the reality of it right now is a lot of my patients I see get better. But then they get sick and they die.

ROBERT BAZELL:  AIDS is caused by a virus which destroys the body's immune system, leading the victims to a variety of rare infections and cancer.  The doctors and nurses here treat those infections but the infections reappear until they are fatal. The staff is trying a number of experimental drugs to try to cure the underlying viral disease, so far without success.

SPEAKER:  At this point none of the interventions that we have been able to do in this clinical setting have served to prolong the life span of a person who has been diagnosed.  It gets to you sometimes, as a cancer specialist; I knew when I entered oncology that I would be dealing with people who were dying. What I didn't realize was that they would be my own age, many of them very similar to me, intelligent people, people that are creative and have contributed to society, and it's devastating when one day after another people die.

ROBERT BAZELL:  The patients here in San Francisco are mostly all homosexual men.  Nationwide three quarters of AIDS victims are gay men.  Talking to these men one hears two themes repeated, one is those that do the best are the ones with the most support from family and friends.

SPEAKER:  You know a lot of people around me pay attention and care.  It makes a big difference.

ROBERT BAZELL:  The other is of being shunned.  AIDS can only be spread by sexual contact or by mixing of blood, not by casual contact.  Many people don't believe that.

SPEAKER:  People might not want to associate with you or they feel like they are going to catch soemthing from you and they kind of take a leper kind of attitude towards you.

ROBERT BAZELL:  When patients get sick they go to the AIDS ward.  The twelve beds here are always full.  Steven Perri is 35 years old.

STEVEN PERRI:  I feel that I will die someday.

In order to put a piece on television you have to have some reason for doing it.  One reason for doing it is to humanize it like we did there, and to involve the audience with individual people which makes them pay more attention.  A lot of times you end up not communicating as many facts as you would like.  I'm going to show you this next piece which I think, because you all know the information that is in there, you will find it boring but it was the result of a lot of discussion that I had with my superiors, and I finally got them to agree to a piece that from a television standpoint, particularly network television, is considered to be very boring.  The idea was that we are just going to have to come out and say things and say them without telling you the life story of somebody or anything else because there seems to be so much hysteria in the country, so much misinformation.  For those of you in clinics the other lesson that you learn in seeing this is that when you let television people in, we use the same pictures over and over again.  What you are going to see in this piece are many of the same people you saw a minute ago but you should realize that these pieces ran two months apart.  If you weren't watching television every night you won't remember it or it wouldn't be so fresh.  So let's go ahead and run this please.

ANCHORMAN:  The many questions about AIDS, just what is this dreaded disease.  What does it do?  Who gets it?  Even though the AIDS epidemic is getting daily new coverage, there remains so much misleading information, so we've asked our science correspondent, Robert Bazell, to take us through these confusing, frightening questions.

ROBERT BAZELL:  What is AIDS?  Acquired Immune Deficiency Syndrome is a disease which destroys the body's immune system. The victim becomes susceptible to a variety of life threatening diseases which are rare in healthy people.

How deadly is it?  AIDS is a fatal disease for which there is no known cure.  On average victims live for about a year and a half from the time that they are diagnosed.  What causes it? AIDS is spread by a virus, infects certain white blood cells. These are pictures of the virus, magnified one hundred thousand times.

How does it spread?  For a person to be infected the virus must enter his bloodstream.  Sexual intercourse, where semen enters the bloodstream is the most common mode of transmission. Researchers know that the disease can be transmitted by homosexual men during intercourse.

They also know that an infected man can transmit the disease to a woman, but it is not certain that an infected woman can transmit it to a man during sex.

Who are the victims?  Homosexual men account for the vast majority of cases.  78 percent of the almost 13,000 AIDS victims in the United States are gay men.  Intravenous drug users make up the next largest group.  They account for 17 percent of the cases.

AIDS is spread by drug users when they share needles. Contaminated blood from an infected person gets injected into the blood stream of the next victim.  Other victims include women, or the wives or lovers of men infected with the virus. They make up about 1 percent of the cases.

Children can be born with AIDS.  157 so far in the U.S.  Their mothers are infected and the children get it from their mother's blood in the womb.  Blood transfusions and blood products can spread AIDS.  260 cases have been reported so far.  But now there is a test to detect the AIDS virus in blood.  Most blood banks use it routinely.  And public health officials believe that this will dramatically reduce the risk from transfusion.

Who can transmit it?  Researchers estimate that one million Americans already have been infected with the AIDS virus. Every infected person will not get the disease.  But every infected person is a potential carrier who can give it to others.

Is the general population at risk?  There is little risk to the general public at this time according to health officials. They do not believe that AIDS will become a major heterosexual venereal disease, such as herpes or gonnorhea.  But the officials warned that the number of AIDS victims continues to rise dramatically.  It is inevitable that there will be more

and more cases among heterosexuals who are not drug users, but who have had sexual contact with an infected person.
Can AIDS be caught by casual contact?  The answer is no.  All the evidence indicates that the virus must get into a person's bloodstream.  AIDS can not be transmitted in the way colds and flu are.  Thousands of doctors, nurses and other health care workers have cared for AIDS patients and not gotten the disease.  Studies of the families of AIDS patients show that the disease does not spread through normal household contact.  So there is one piece of good news about this awful disease.

We have two more to go.  I am attempting to give you an idea of the range of the things that we have done.  For a long time, I have been trying to get into Africa to do a piece.  It certainly wasn't an easy task.  I think that I am the only American television correspondent to get into Africa and when we did, it became in retrospect almost a circus.  At the time it was expensive, difficult, and we were promised certain things by governments, who then reneged on their promises once we got there.

We had a stringer who was working for us in Nairobi who had a visit from the secret police in the middle of the night, tore up our apartment, threatened her life all because she was asking questions about AIDS.  That was the level of the attitudes of governments in Africa.

ANCHORMAN:  There is one more issue associated with AIDS and it demonstrates the seriousness of this epidemic.

Of all the people who have been diagnosed as having AIDS nearly half of them, about seven thousand altogether have died.  There is evidence tonight of the rapid threat of AIDS on heterosexuals in Africa.  The scientific studies will be presented at a conference on AIDS in Brussels.  They show the virus as spreading much faster in Africa than anywhere else and they indicate that up to seven percent of the adult population of two countries, Zaire and Congo, men and women may be carrying this disease.

To illustrate the rapid spread of AIDS in Africa, NBC science correspondent, Robert Bazell, visited one part of Tanzania.

ROBERT BAZELL:  Serina Obustum is coming to the local hospital in Bacova, Tanzania, because she fears she is suffering from the new illness appearing in this region.

Local people call it Slim Disease because the victims lose weight rapidly.  Dr. Clinton Amray Coumay takes a blood sample on the 23 year old woman.  When it is sent away to be analyzed he is certain that he will prove that Serina will have Slim Disease,  what we call AIDS.

More and more AIDS cases are filling the beds of the hospital here.  Bacova is the center of the Cagera region of Tanzania on the shore of Lake Victoria, most of the Ugandan border.

Here is Cagera Province.  There were no AIDS cases before 1983, now the disease is widespread.  Doctors say many victims don't even seek treatment because they have learned that there is no cure.

Dr. Amray Coumay, with few resources, tries to help those who
do appear. But it is likely Serina will soon become as sick as
19 year old Padatoni.

SPEAKER: This is a difficult patient. Really all of them can
stay for 6 months or so and then they expire.

ROBERT BAZELL: Half of the AIDS victims here are women.
Talking to them, the doctors have learned that most are
single. Most say they have had several sexual partners. 33
year old Felix Garanea is a typical male victim. He is married
and the doctors suspect he visits prostitutes, mostly on visits
to Uganda and Kenya.

The doctors have no doubt that AIDS is a heterosexual disease.
Some American and European doctors said it originated in
Africa; this angers African doctors.

SPEAKER: It is not very important to know where the disease
originated. What is important to know is that we have a
problem and to look for ways of solving it.

ROBERT BAZELL: Tanzania is the only African country to admit
it has a problem with AIDS. Others fear loss of tourists and
trade. The Tanzania doctors say they need help.

SPEAKER: We need to devote time to this problem and to educate
our people on the modes of transmission of this disease and
hope that by prevention we might check the spread of this
disease.

ROBERT BAZELL: For now the chance of stopping the disease is
slim. Unless researchers discover something unique about AIDS
in Africa, it remains possible that AIDS will spread among
heterosexuals in other parts of the world. Robert Bazell, NBC
News, Bacova, Tanzania.

I have shown you some of my travels now to several places, to
San Francisco, to Haiti, to Africa. The last piece I am going to
show you is a piece that I should have done a long time before I
did it.

It involved traveling, literally, eight blocks from my home to
do this spot. I live in Manhattan. I will show that to you now
and my concluding remarks.

ANCHORMAN: There is a new concern among AIDS researchers that
drug addicts not homosexuals now pose a greater threat for
spreading the disease. NBC correspondent, Robert Bazell
tonight reports on the deadly connection between AIDS and drug
addiction.

ROBERT BAZELL: Young addicts injecting heroin into their veins
in an empty lot on the lower East Side of Manhattan.

First they dissolve the drug. As they inject it they pull
large amounts of blood into the syringe to make certain that
they get all the heroin into their bodies. It is because so

much blood is involved that the widespread practice of sharing needles has spread AIDS rapidly among drug users.
One infected addict leaves his blood containing the virus in the needle and the next one to use the needle gets the AIDS virus into his bloodstream.

SPEAKER:  I had heard about AIDS.  I knew very little about it and I knew that drug users could get it, but you know, I used that old phrase, I'll never get it.

ROBERT BAZELL:  Cheryl Accasella is one of the more than 28,000 people in this country who has gotten AIDS from sharing needles.  But that number is just a beginning.  Public Health officials estimate that hundreds of thousands of people have been infected with the AIDS virus from drug use.

No one knows how many will get sick, but they can all infect others.  Almost all of the hundreds of children born with AIDS or AIDS related illnesses have been victims of drug use.  Most have mothers that are drug users, while the rest are the wives or lovers of drug users.

These addicts know about AIDS, they say they try to avoid sharing their needles and syringes, what they call their works.

SPEAKER:  I use a brand new set every time.

ROBERT BAZELL:  But addicts admit that when they are sick from withdrawal, they forget the precautions.

SPEAKER:  You don't think about no AIDS, or nothing, when you're sick, you get some works from somebody and you get off . . .

ROBERT BAZELL:  Because of that attitude, officials believe that drug users present the greatest danger for the spread of AIDS in the future.

SPEAKER:  They are clearly a major threat for transmission through heterosexual contact.

ROBERT BAZELL:  Health officials have suggested various plans for educating addicts about the dangers of AIDS.  The drug users have always been one of the most difficult to educate. It is obvious that a daily dose of heroin is far more important to them than fear of AIDS.  Robert Bazell, NBC News, New York.

I hope that these examples serve to focus at least on some of the things that we want to talk about in this presentation.  I conclude by saying that I have regarded AIDS, as by far, the most important story I have ever covered in my ten years at NBC, my 15 years as a scientist, the most important thing I have ever dealt with since my training as a scientist.  I may not have approached it with the existential viewpoints that Nathan described, I'm sorry that I have not thought about it along the way but we tried to do a good job.  I certainly hope that we will do a better job in the future. Thank you.

COMMENTS

<u>Jim Bunn</u> (Reporter, KPIX-TV, San Francisco)

I have been reporting on the AIDS epidemic for three years. I am a general assignments reporter. I do not have a science background. I am probably more like the reporter many of you have had to deal with when you confront the press. Most of the people covering the epidemic in the local press are generalists, instant experts, that is what we are required to be.

About a year and a half ago, the management of the television station that I work for decided that in San Francisco we needed to do more than just have someone in the newsroom who reported most of the AIDS stories. They took a rather unique, (certainly in my 13 years in the business), unprecedented step of giving a general assignments reporter one day off each week from the street to do nothing but research AIDS.

So my reading list changed from US News and World Report, Time, Newsweek, People, etc. to MMWR, JAMA, New England Journal of Medicine and Lancet, etc.

I also used the time to visit with people like Dean Echenberg, Don Abrams, Paul Volberding, and Merv Silverman to take what I describe as AIDS 101. It was patently obvious when I began reporting in San Francisco three years ago that I was in way over my head on a subject that was going to be around for a long, long time. I needed to get on it as quickly as I could.

These people were my teachers and brought me up-to-speed and got me to a level where I could at least discuss the story and the epidemic with some intelligence to others who are fighting this epidemic.

I kept hearing a recurring theme about education and I kept hearing the hue and cry from people that not enough was being done. And as we are here today to discuss the media's role in this epidemic it became apparent to me that this was going to be one of those rare circumstances where I was part of the story, not just reporting it. I took this feeling to the people who run my television station and my company, Westinghouse Broadcasting, and I said, "we are a business entity in a community that is in the midst of a public health crisis. We should do something because we are a mouthpiece to the general population, a population that has yet not seen the virus spread to the degree that it has in the high risk groups."

There is a moral imperative here but the people who run the television stations are business people and they don't function, they are not paid to function, at a level of moral imperatives. They are paid to deal with the bottom line. And we were able to convince the people who run the business of television that there was a way to get involved with the public health crisis and have it be good for business.

With the premise that the best defense against AIDS is
information, we started a station wide project called AIDS Lifeline
and the title was something that we agonized over and it is no
accident. The premise of my pitch to the bosses was, yes, all of
the negative associations people have with AIDS could be a risk to
our business and to our image in the community. However, the
reason that there is a negative association because people are
scared to death of this damn thing.

"If we can do something to allay that fear, they will like us.
They will feel better about us, that's good for business. Image is
very important in television." The AIDS Lifeline project got
started very quickly with Dr. Merv Silverman on board as our staff
consultant to make sure that we had our act together. He also lent
credibility to the correctness of what we were saying and to the
degree of our commitment. What we did and are doing involves a
series of public service announcements with celebrities from
Hollywood, a series of special inserts on the talk shows involving
Dr. Silverman and occasionally myself on the programming side. We
have also produced two documentaries, one of which has been
syndicated around the country to fifteen cities, a documentary we
found later to be the first of its kind in that it dealt with the
overall aspect of the AIDS epidemic. We were dealing not just with
the medicine and the science but we were dealing with the ethical
questions, the social questions, the money, how government is
responding to it, etc. That documentary has been requested to be
used as a teaching tape by better than 200 private and public
institutions in this country from the Baltimore Fire Department to
DuPont Chemical. Now we didn't do this program with that thought
in mind but it's some evidence for the need that does exist and the
desire that exists in this country for information.

What we will continue to do is to do what we can in our AIDS
Lifeline reports to advance the story. The reports that appear on
the regular newscast are not one and a half to three minutes in
length, they are more five, six, seven, eight, ten minutes in
length. More of a mini documentary if you will. And what we have
found is that we can give an appropriate amount of depth and
substance to the stories as you saw in some of Bob's work.

In addition to the public service announcements, we have
printed literature that is very specific in its language. It was
produced by the San Francisco AIDS Foundation which has been doing
this for quite a while. They know how to handle printed literature
better than a television station does. It was done in concert with
the San Francisco Health Department.

What happened with the public service announcements is they
encouraged people to get the printed literature. We had an initial
printing of 40,000. Now there are close to a million in print, in
five languages, around the world. This is without any kind of
marketing effort. Dr. Fineberg referred yesterday to the Madison
Avenue approach for a national education program for AIDS risk
reduction. I couldn't agree with him more. What we have with our
experience in San Francisco is a small example of how it can be
done in a very rudimentary way and it's something that deserves
serious consideration and discussion. Thank you.

**Tony Whitehead** (Chairperson, Terrence Higgins Trust, London, England)

The Terrence Higgins Trust is an equivalent to the GMHC but a lot smaller, but I think that if I describe very briefly how it was set-up and how we run you will recognize many features in common. Three years ago we were six people in my front room in an apartment in London. We are now three hundred volunteers and yet we only still have two full-time paid staff. We hope to increase that very soon.

Like GMHC, we were originally solely composed of gay men, many of us experienced in gay community organizations and that's really our particular background. We have, like the organizations in America, diversified since then and tried very hard to provide support and education services that will serve the community at large.

Naturally with the resources that we have, it is very limited. My major concern and one of the major concerns of the Trust is education. That is why I was very glad to come along here today. I do not put myself up as an expert on the role of the media, but as a critic of the way in which the media has worked. I think it is fair to say in Britain, at the present time and indeed over the last three years, it has been as bad if not worse than the media that you have in America. Indeed I was extremely impressed by the television reports that we saw because in terms of the clarity of explaining the issues, they are very good indeed.

We have about three national documentaries on BBC and ITV in Britain which could hold their head up with that but very little else. In terms of general newspaper coverage, we have very little.

I don't look to the media to get over the education or the preventive messages. I believe that the media has its particular role to play in society, whether or not it plays that role very well is a moot point but it is in the business of presenting the news, and news and education are not, I believe, compatible. We are certainly, constantly concerned that the media has fudged the issue. If I could just pick up on the last of those TV programs describing drug users as the danger because it's through them that AIDS will spread to the general population. That kind of terminology where the media has looked at disenfranchised groups, such as gay men and drug users and described them as a danger rather than clearly focusing on the disease itself, has reinforced public prejudices. But my major concern, in terms of education, is for a clear and unambiguous education campaign that I don't think that newspapers are going to put out. It is for groups like the Trust, and groups such as we've heard about in San Francisco and New York, to put over those clear educational messages in unambiguous language is not news but it is very important.

We have at our disposal walking around this part of New York and seeing Madison Avenue enormous resources. I disagree with Nathan Fain in his description of the way in which gay men are alienated from authority as being a major obstacle. Speaking as a gay man myself, I understand the presence of alienation and suspicion of authority which actually puts us as the problem, the disparity between innocent and guilty people with AIDS which we see

all the time in the media.  But gay men, as anybody else, are
influenced into buying a particular brand of cigarettes and liquor
and clothes, cars.  Therefore, I feel that what we should look for
in terms of prevention on AIDS is not necessarily to put the
responsibility solely on the backs of the media.  If they could
have presented this news more clearly presented the arguments more
clearly than they have done and to take out some of the motives and
misleading terminology which they use, and to regard gay men as
profit to society and not the problem of AIDS, that would be
enough.  What we need in terms of education I believe, is to look
to the skills of advertisers who are particularly the best people,
in terms of persuading us in the behavior changes to say, that AIDS
is not casually caught.  It's a very difficult disease to catch.  I
think we should look to those skills in order to get those messages
across.

Now, at the present time in Britain, we are singularly failing
to do that because of being starved of resources.  The volunteer
sector in Britian which is the sector that is being most concerned
with education, work so far as we see with 1.5 million pounds.  A
very small amount in money, indeed.  Two and a half million pounds
is being earmarked for education so far but it is not being spent.

What we have seen in Britain in terms of education work in the
newspapers is two one-page newspaper pieces going out in our
National Press.  Both of those were compromised and are too far on
the side of political expediency and public delicacy.  Their use of
language is obscure.  We had terms such as intimate kissing may be
a danger, God knows  what that is, I still don't know whether it's
how you kiss or which bit of the body you kiss.

We had rectal intercourse.  How many people understand
terminology like rectal intercourse.  Any intercourse would have
been an improvement and fucking would have been a lot better in the
context of Britain.

We need to communicate these issues clearly, we need to
communicate them unambiguously.  Looking to the media in terms of
its presentation of the news is only a small part of that.  Until
we receive the kinds of funding necessary to develop the expertise
in advertising; until they realize that embarrassments and
difficulties are a necessary cost in order that we may save many
thousands of lives in Britian, I am very pessimistic that we are
actually going to be able to mount a sensible national education
campaign.

The Trust would be willing to do that work, to do the
government's dirty work.  We have to work within the system, we
have to work with newspapers as they are and understand what their
role is.  We have to work with governments and political parties as
they are.  We are willing to do the dirty work even though it is
their responsibility.  However, we can not do it without the money
and without the goodwill and help from people like my colleague
Andrew Veitch.  That is my major cry and that is where I am coming
from.  I don't put myself up here as a media expert, I have a job
to do and the job is AIDS prevention.  We have to communicate to
many of the high risk groups.  We have many ways of reaching them.
What we need is money, what we need is backing and that's what we
are lacking.

**Michael Callen** (New York State AIDS Advisory Council, Member, People with AIDS Coalition)

I guess I was invited onto this panel to be the "bad boy"--to argue that the media has been, by and large, grossly irresponsible in terms of its AIDS reporting. That certainly is my position; but I'm not here to beat up on Robert or Jim--two men who take this issue seriously enough to be here and open themselves up to critical scrutiny. And, of course, there has been some exceptional AIDS reporting.

But on the whole, it is my view that the seriousness and complexity of the AIDS story--it's political, medical, social and human consequences--have exposed in stark relief many of the problems of the American media in general. In other words, although TV and print have done a particularly terrible job of reporting about AIDS, I'm not so sure how much more terrible it has been than, say, its reporting on terrorism or the Reagan presidency or Chernobyl or crack.

I will spare you the many examples of shoddy reporting and provide, instead, the one I consider to be the most damning. As you may recall, President Johnson was hounded out of the presidency in large part by the media's relentless, probing reportage concerning his handling of the Vietnam war. This was as it should have been, because American boys were dying. And yet with estimates that more Americans may die from AIDS by 1990 than died during the entire Vietnam War, President Reagan did not publicly utter the word "AIDS" until the Rock Hudson story broke. In other words, he was permitted by the media to go through an entire first term and a bitter election campaign without ever once being questioned about his administration's handling of the most serious health crisis within recent memory. This is a rather scorching indictment of American journalism.

The main problem, it seems to me, is a general distrust of the public's intelligence--expressed by the 15-second bit mentality. Frankly, there are many complex ideas which just can't be boiled down to a 15-second bit--particularly when it comes to a story as complicated as AIDS. Generally, it seems the media either doesn't risk doing complex stories or finds those so-called "experts" who "come across well" on TV: who can smile for the camera and seem to be believable or reassuring. Whether these "experts" are in fact telling the truth seems to be less important than style. The scandal of the U.S. theft of credit from France for first describing a certain retrovirus associated with AIDS; the apparent misclassification of HIV as a member of the HTLV-III family rather than the visna virus family; and Heckler's bizarre and glib prediction of a vaccine within a year demonstrate to me that when it comes to AIDS, usually skeptical journalists are all too eager to uncritically believe what they're told by the government.

Now, it's fashionable to huff and puff about how stupid the parents in Queens were. But I think their fears, though misguided, were entirely understandable given what they've been told about AIDS by the media. If I faced, almost nightly, news reports that a killer virus was on the loose--that a single "unlucky" contact could lead to AIDS and death--I'd be scared too.

126

And, I hasten to point out, the media is certainly not in a position to throw stones at the folks from Queens. Currently, at several TV stations, sound and camera crews have the right to refuse to work on an AIDS story and, I understand, several TV unions have succeeded in getting higher pay--a "combat differential"--for those willing to "risk" pinning a microphone on me.

And then there's all this equivocation about "casual contact"--this squeamish unwillingness to speak frankly about fucking and condoms and IV drug use. We may all agree that it's silly and Puritanical. But we don't often state the blunt fact that, in this case, such silliness is killing people!

I've made it my business to encourage skepticism. I consider skepticism not only healthy, but crucial--because the stakes are so high. I'm a fan of Sir Karl Popper, whose view is that we can never know for sure if something is absolutely true. But, he proposed, we can know what is false. And we approximate scientific truth by our inability to disprove a proposition. Regarding the virtual non-debate about the etiology of AIDS, HTLV-III has become a matter of faith--almost a religion. To question its central role in AIDS is heresy--and a guarantee of no funding and ridicule. But the history of science is littered with orthodoxies--believed at one time by a majority--which were proved wrong.

I'll end by saying that if I believed everything I was told--if I believed that tiresome boilerplate that AIDS is "100 percent fatal"--then I'd probably be dead by now. If I didn't arm myself with information--with diverse views, I would be unable to defend myself from the madness and gibberish which daily assaults those of us who have AIDS.


Andrew Veitch (Medical Correspondent, The Guardian, London, England)

Hello, I'm glad to hear that the American media occasionally makes mistakes, from the little bit of American reporting that I have seen you are a hell of a lot better than us, which is a pretty sad comment on English newspapers.

I used to say that you could cure the media's problems with AIDS quite simply by getting us information, by throwing open the door, by giving what was happening clear and straight. We would retail it, and the fear and loathing that goes with ignorance would be dispelled.

I was wrong. I found out I was wrong last week when I helped the Royal Society in London to organize a symposium on AIDS for the Press. The idea was to tell everyone what was happening so you would have good, factual, reporting. The next day, my own paper, The Guardian, to my eternal shame, gave AIDS to the Gambia. That was slightly embarrassing for us, very embarrassing for the Gambia, and very embarrassing for the Royal Society. I spent the rest of the week trying to correct the mistake. There are no cases of AIDS in the Gambia.

What's gone wrong? I think in general you, as doctors, have got through to us, the front line reporters, the guys who have been covering AIDS day in day out for three years or so. I think we have got an idea what's going on-as far as anyone has. We have become a little discriminatory in whom we talk to. I think we now know whom we can trust to give us honest and reliable information, and we know whom to avoid.

But I think that we, in turn, have failed to get through to the people who really make the papers-the editors, the sub-editors, the guys who decide what goes in the pages, the guys who write the headlines that you hate so much.

Sometimes I wonder exactly what we're up against. I think that one answer, to put it simply, may be sexual hangups. You have to be pretty queer to work on a newspaper, you have to be very queer to work on a newspaper at night, and the result is that you end up with a lot of macho hairy-ass guys who are terrified to admit that one time in their dim and distant past they may have had a homosexual relationship.

We are very hung up. I think that it has become manifest in the way that we have coped with the AIDS story. It is always treated as something dirty, something that is happening to them out there, whether they are gays or drug addicts or prostitutes.

I don't think doctors are protected from those hang ups. But you can mask your hang ups when you go into print-at least when you write in the New England Journal of Medicine or the Lancet. You don't have to write "anal intercourse" if you don't want to, you can write "rectal intercourse." Though for some reason I have never heard anyone use the term "receptive rectal intercourse." I get very confused about these things.

Now we on The Guardian have a funny sort of system. I've been trying to use the words "anal intercourse" for two years now and I can't get them in the paper. The usual reason I am given is that it's just too boring. So I try the words "receptive anal intercourse" to get a bit of flavor into it, and my editors say, "What's that?" I think next time we will try "buggery" and see what happens.

We have another little rule. You can get "fuck" into The Guardian as long as it is in the arts pages and the theatre reviews and it's artistically justified. So you can say "fuck" to your readers over their corn flakes in the morning, but you can't say "anal intercourse". It's a bit of wonderful hypocrisy.

How do we get over that? How do we report the story if we can't use the necessary language? God knows. Last night at dinner I heard one guy who I think might help to break through the barriers, to force us to realise we can write about homosexuals without hangups. It was Bishop Paul Moore. His was one of the most courageous speeches that I have heard. It was the sort of speech that forced you to challenge your fears, to break those very old and silly attitudes. Maybe when more Church leaders and politicians follow his example, we'll get somewhere.

Keynote Address:  AIDS in the United Kingdom

E. Donald Acheson, D.M., F.R.C.P., F.F.C.M., M.F.O.M.
Chief Medical Officer, Department of Health and Social Security,
London, England

KEYNOTE ADDRESS:  AIDS IN THE UNITED KINGDOM

E. Donald Acheson, D.M., F.R.C.P., F.F.C.M., M.F.O.M.

Chief Medical Officer
Department of Health and Social Security
London, England

A sound public health policy has to be based on scientific
knowledge about the disease in question.  So I am going to start
with a few words which place the situation about AIDS in the United
Kingdom in context and in perspective.  The principal
epidemiological effects of the outbreak of HIV infection are well
known to everyone here.  The key features which make control
difficult are that the infection is spread predominantly, at any
rate in the United Kingdom, by sexual transmission and that there is
a period of infectivity which lasts months, years, or is possibly
life-long in persons who are usually unaware that they are
infectious.  Of course percutaneous and perinatal transmission also
occurs.  And if we link these features with the facts that the
infection is potentially fatal, that there is no effective
vaccination or treatment in sight, and that the groups most at risk
are to a substantial extent stigmatized and alienated, we have a
terrible spectacle and an immensely complex set of problems to solve.

In the United Kingdom the first case of AIDS was reported at the
end of 1981 and the number of cases detected by national
surveillance has subsequently increased rapidly.  But the number of
cases reported is very small relative to the United States.  We have
had, in all, 375 cases of AIDS up to the end of April 1986 of which
80% were reported from London and most of the remainder from a few
large urban centers in England.  Predictions using two different
approaches suggest that in the United Kingdom in 1988, there may be
about 2,000 new cases.  But this estimate has wide confidence
limits.  In recent months, there has been some evidence of
flattening of the rate of increase of reported cases.  The reasons
for this are uncertain.  Up to the 30th of December, 1985, the
United Kingdom ranked 9th in AIDS incidence among 23 reporting
European countries.

Allowing that about half of the cases are dead and about 1/3 to
a half of the living cases are in hospital at any time there are
probably between 60 and 90 patients suffering from AIDS in hospital
in the United Kingdom today.  The majority of these are in
London.

In the United Kingdom, as in this country, the first AIDS cases were reported among male homosexuals and these have contributed by far the largest proportion of all our cases, in fact just under 90 percent. But in contrast to the United States, the illness among drug abusers has so far been rare. In the United Kingdom in 1984, the annual incidence rate of AIDS among single men over 15 years of age was approximately 1 per 100,000 compared with 14 per 100,000 in the United States. In greater London the incidence was about 5 per 100,000 as compared with between 260 and 340 per 100,000 in New York and San Francisco.

The average prevalence figure for 1984-5 among male homosexuals attenders at genitourinary clinics was 21 percent. In drug abusers the comparable figure is lower, about 10 percent, but the recent report of prevalence rates in excess of 50 percent in drug abusers in Edinburgh, Scotland, is an extremely ominous development. It is estimated that there may be between 800 and 1,000 seropositive drug abusers in the east of Scotland, with both sexes affected almost equally and, of course, some infected babies have already been born.

The prevalence of antibody in hemophiliacs does not appear to have increased since 1984 when heat treated factor VIII and IX generally became available. The reported prevalence of antibodies in female sexual partners of hemophiliacs is about the same in Britain as in the U.S. Our numbers are very small, 7 percent based on 5 out of 75 cases.

Although there is no information about the prevalence of HIV antibody in the general population in the U.K. in strict epidemiological terms, data from compulsory screening of donations from the national blood transfusion service suggests that it is very low. Among just under 1 1/2 million donations from apparently healthy male and female blood donors most of whom are in the sexually active age group (persons belonging to high risk groups have been asked not to donate blood), only 32 confirmed positive tests have been found. That's about 0.02 per 100,000. Of the 32 almost all were found subsequently to actually have been at risk, either homosexual males or drug abusers. And of the 32, it is interesting that 30 are male and 2 female, although the prevalence of blood donations in the U.K. is approximately equal between the two sexes.

Although blood donors are not representative of adults in general, this suggests that at present in the U.K. the prevalence of specific antibodies outside the risk groups is low and that the infection remains largely confined to those groups.

It's difficult to reconcile the data from this country, the United Kingdom and Europe on the one hand with those from certain areas of Central Africa on the other. I don't want to go into this in any detail but the position we take from the public health point of view about heterosexual transmission in the United Kingdom is that prudence dictates that the sexually active population as a whole should be regarded as possibly at risk and should receive practical advice about how the infection can be avoided.

Now let us turn to the question of public policy which must be directed, first of all, at the control of the spread of the infection, and secondly, at provision of care for those who are affected.

In the absence of an effective vaccine or antiviral agent, the means available to control the spread of infection are strictly limited. The most important is, first of all, education of the public about how the infection is and is not spread, including advice about the avoidance of infection and safe sex. Secondly, advice to infected persons to help them avoid infecting others is crucial. Thirdly, provision of a safe supply of blood for transfusion and of products derived from blood is necessary to limit the spread of infection.

As far as education is concerned, it will be necessary for the programs to be tailored both to those actually at risk or at high risk and those potentially at risk. As you will have heard from some of the remarks yesterday, in the United Kingdom a program of public education sponsored by the government has begun. It's a three pronged program. It involves not only special programs designed to meet the needs of declared male homosexuals and persons who abuse drugs by injection, but also material directed to the population as a whole. As far as the general campaign is concerned, the first objective is to reduce unnecessary fears by disspelling myths and by providing accurate information about HIV and AIDS. A general campaign is also required to inform undeclared homosexual and bisexual men who do not read the gay press or attend gay clubs or discos and to provide information for all sexually active men and women. Adolescents must also be given information about the infection and how it is spread so that, for example, they become aware of the new grave risks associated with experiments in injecting drugs.

During March and April of this year full page AIDS prevention advertisements were published in all the national newspapers in the UK. In all, probably some 100 million copies of the ad were printed. It covered a pretty comprehensive range of subjects. At the top it indicated that it comes from the four doctors who are chief medical officers of the four countries in the United Kingdom. Among the headings included in the ad were, What is AIDS? How is AIDS spread? How is it not spread? It made a statement that AIDS not only affects homosexuals. It attempted to talk also about safe sex and risky sex. It said that using a sheath reduces the risk of AIDS and other diseases. Sexual intercourse with an infected person is risky, any act that damages the penis, vagina, anus or mouth is dangerous. It went on to say that AIDS is not spread through normal contact with other people, that AIDS is not spread by objects touched by infected people, that blood transfusions are safe and so on. It gave a telephone number from which you can get more explicit advice and also an address from which you can get a much more explicit pamphlet.

Now in retrospect I can tell you that those advertisements caused no criticism with respect to being too explicit. They caused no shock or horror from the right wing or from the churches or anything of that sort. They were criticized to some extent for being insufficiently explicit and there was one other criticism, and I have to tell you that I received in all about 12 letters of criticism about this, despite about 100 million copies of the ad. It did not clearly indicate that there are gradations of risk. For example, between a homosexual encounter in London where perhaps 30 percent of the people are seropositive and a heterosexual encounter in London where the risk might be 3 or 4 or 5 orders of magnitude less. It didn't clearly state that. There was a reason for that:

in addition to the possibility of shock and horror about explicit material going through everybody's mailbox on Sunday in the whole land, there was also anxiety lest we should create a gay backlash in any way, and the thing was very carefully looked at from that point of view.  It didn't produce any sort of backlash of that sort.  And I leave you to judge whether, or to what extent, this was an act of some political courage.

Of course, it is a first step.  Now we know, or the ministers with whom I work know, that they are not going to be attacked for being too explicit and shocking everybody and letting children read about nasty things.  We are in a position to go ahead and we are planning a campaign which will take us forward.

In addition, a pamphlet is also going to all schools for teachers to explain to them how they should handle children who are HIV positive and inviting them to include information about AIDS in sex education.  The special campaigns directed particularly at the gay community and to people who abuse drugs by injection are being dealt with through the voluntary agencies and the health education councils.  Education to professionals, free booklets about AIDS have gone out to all doctors in the country and one has gone out to nurses.  There are also instructions which are directed to all health care workers in hospitals handling specimens.

There also has to be public policy on counseling.  Trained counselors should be available in all genitourinary medicine clinics to advise patients in all risk groups, their partners, patients in whom a test for HIV is indicated, and those who have specific antibodies.

The essence of the advice is to avoid abusing drugs by injection, to use safe sexual practices, reduce the number of partners, and, where the patient or partner is at risk, to use a condom for penetrative intercourse.  Advice about the risks of perinatal transmission of infection to children should also be available to women at risk of HIV.  Each of the 192 health districts in England has been asked to formulate a plan to deal with both prevention and treatment and these plans are coming into the Department of Health for scrutiny.

With the prime objective of rendering blood transfusion as safe as possible, tests for specific antibodies to HIV infection were introduced by the National Blood Transfusion Service and made generally available throughout the U.K. in October 1985.  And I have mentioned the results of the first 1 1/2 million tests.

Opinions differ as to whether in addition it is appropriate to use such tests as a tool in the control of spread of infection by sexual transmission.  One view is that these tests should not be offered on a routine basis or promoted as a means of control of infection because there is no effective treatment which can be offered to infected patients who are free of symptoms and because it can be detrimental to a person to know that he or she has a positive test such as in connection with and application for life insurance. Furthermore the advice, namely to avoid unsafe practices and reduce partners is the same whether a person has a positive or negative test.  Others, both in the medical profession and outside, take the opposite view.  They consider the tests for HIV antibodies are an important means of controlling spread and should therefore be promoted by campaigns designed to encourage all those who have been at risk to come forward. The object would be to ensure that as many as possible of all those in the population that have been infected would be advised how to minimize the risk of transmitting the infection to others.

The fact that infected women can pass HIV to a subsequently conceived child is a point that should be taken into consideration in this discussion. Because it follows that men and women who have specific antibodies to HIV have a responsibility which men and women who are negative do not. A knowledge of the result of a positive test gives them an opportunity to make an informed choice. This suggests the HIV antibody testing should be encouraged at least in genitourinary medicine clinics for patients who may be bisexual and for women who are partners of men at risk and for drug abusers.

The second point is more speculative. Is that patient in a risk group more likely to change his behavior if he knows whether he is HIV positive or negative or if he or she does not know? This question urgently requires an answer. If any change of sexual behavior in the direction of less risk is more likely when a person knows whether he is seropositive or negative, there would be a case for promoting such a test. In the United Kingdom, at present, except in the National Blood Transfusion Service where it is carried out on all donations, the use of the test is not the subject of promotion but it is generally available for use at the discretion of doctor and patient. It is difficult for government to take other than a neutral line on this issue when the medical profession and other representatives of the gay community are divided amongst themselves about it. The idea that testing for specific antibodies should be a pre-condition for the issue of a visa to enter a country has been rejected by most countries including the United Kingdom, although it is the policy of the Saudi Arabian government.

In western countries, by far the most important non-sexual means of transmission is among drug abusers who share infected equipment. There are wide differences in the prevalence of HIV in drug abusers in different localities which, if explained, may point to preventive action. I have mentioned the problem we have in Edinburgh, for example. These require urgent investigation. Perinatal transmission of infection is an important risk among seropositive drug abusers. At the moment we are not convinced within the U.K. that the provision of syringes and needles to people who take illegal drugs by injection would be helpful in controlling the spread of HIV infection. There are arguments in both directions. Some physicians and others think that such provision would increase the spread of the disease; others think it would reduce it. But the matter is not closed and is under urgent consideration.

No plan for control of communicable disease is complete without effective epidemiological surveillance. The scheme followed in the U.K. consists of doctors being invited to report cases of AIDS to our communicable disease surveillance center in strict confidence. This is not legal notification; it is doctor-to-doctor, professional, if you like, arrangement. It has worked well although it has no force of law. It is strictly confidential. In recent months, confidential reporting of positive HIV antibody tests to CDSC has begun. It is controversial whether it is acceptable to test sera from unknown persons without their consent for public health purposes. Looked at strictly from the public health point of

view, it would be extremely helpful to have information about the
prevalence of specific antibodies from unbiased, systematic samples
from people so the course of the epidemic could be followed.  But
the medical profession and its legal advisors have not made up its
mind about the ethics nor have the people in general, and in these
circumstances, it is not possible for government to take a lead.

A word about confidentiality and other social issues relating to
AIDS.  The success of a plan for the control of the spread of HIV
infection is linked with a number of social issues.  Prime among
these is the question of confidentiality.  Experience has shown that
most people that have been exposed to a sexually transmitted disease
wish the fact of any consultation to be kept strictly confidential.
To meet this need in the United Kingdom a system of free walk-in
clinics where anonymity is guaranteed was set up in response to
public anxiety about the rise and incidence of syphilis and
gonorrhea during the first World War in 1917.  This unique system
which includes the provision that clinical records are locked away
separate from the main hospital records has worked well and is
protected by special regulation.  As a result, no one in the U.K.
need feel that he has to become a blood donor to find out whether he
is seropositive.

The regulations relating to confidentiality require that when an
infection has been sexually transmitted, employees of a health
authority may not disclose information to persons not involved in
the treatment of the patient without the patient's consent.  In
seropositive cases, the doctor will advise the patient how to avoid
transmitting the infection to others and also recommend that the
sexual partner or partners should be told.  The doctor has
discretion to inform a third party to prevent the spread of
infection.  The principle which underlies these strict rules
governing disclosure is that unless confidence is guaranteed
patients will not wish to come forward for diagnosis and
counseling.  This will tend to drive the condition underground and
increase the risk of spread.

Other issues which are being considered in a number of countries
are the control of spread in residential institutions such as
prisons and in the armed forces.  In the United Kingdom, recruits to
the armed forces are not screened, unlike the United States.

The implication for persons with positive tests who subsequently
wish to take out life insurance policies or mortgages needs to be
considered and is a problem in our country as it is in yours.  Some
organizations within the gay community recommend that homosexual men
should not come forward for testing until arrangements have been
made which ensure that persons with positive tests are not subject
to financial detriment.  The government has set up an
interdepartmental ministerial group to consider these and other
issues.

Finally, a few words before my concluding remarks:  First of
all, stigmatization.  Stigma is an enemy of effective public health
policy.  We only have to think of leprosy, tuberculosis and
epilepsy.  It should be an object of government policy to do nothing
to increase stigmatization.  For example, government should be
extremely careful to do nothing which would produce backlash.  Also,
notification and quarantine have no place in the control of HIV.

Provision for care. The National Health Service is 100 percent public funded from central, what you would call federal, funds. So the question of the cost of care is not a major issue. We reckon that the direct health cost of an AIDS case is between 30 and 60 thousand pounds. Some extra money has been found for the areas of London where most of the cases are being looked after.

In conclusion, I have reviewed the epidemiology of HIV infection in the U.K. from the point of view of control of spread of infection and I have tried to place the outbreak in context with those in other countries. Judging by the reported cases, the incidence of AIDS in the U.K. is at present substantially lower that in the United States and a number of European countries. In the U.K. the patterns of incidence of AIDS and of seroprevalence resembles those in other Western countries and differ from those reported from Central Africa.

In the U.K. as in the U.S.A. the infection is at present largely confined to homosexual and bisexual men, hemophiliacs, persons who abuse drugs by injection and the sexual partners of these groups. Nevertheless, as transmission can occur as a result of vaginal intercourse, public health policy must take into account the fact that heterosexual men and women may also be at risk. In the absence of a vaccine or effective antiviral agent, public education to help people avoid risky sexual behavior and drug abuse is the mainstay of a policy for control of spread of infection.

Such programs must meet the different needs of the general population of the groups particularly at risk and of adolescents. They must also include facts about how HIV is and is not transmitted. Practical advice on its avoidance and advice to affected persons to help them avoid infecting others. A policy in relation to the control of spread of infection among drug abusers is also needed and is under consideration. If the use of serotesting is to be promoted for the control of infection, there will need to be prior agreement about its efficacy. People who have been at risk are unlikely to come forward in large numbers unless they feel confident that confidentiality will be preserved and that the problem of financial detriment to seropositive people has been solved.

It is important that no measures are taken which will have the effect of increasing the degree of stigmatization suffered by affected persons and patients with AIDS. Because it is more difficult to control the spread of a communicable disease in stigmatized and alienated groups there is no place for formal notification by law or quarantine in this condition.

Thank you.

Session E: AIDS and Economics: An International Perspective

Participants

Speakers

J. B. Brunet, M.D.
Director, World Health Organization Collaborating Center on AIDS,
Paris, France

Rashi Fein, Ph.D.
Professor, Economics of Medicine, Harvard Medical School

Panelists

Daniel Fox, Ph.D.
Director, New York State Center for Assessing Health Services,
State University of New York at Stony Brook

Fakhry Assaad, M.D., M.P.H.
Director, Division of Communicable Diseases, World Health
Organization, Geneva, Switzerland

Victor Fuchs, Ph.D.
Professor of Economics, Stanford University, Research Associate,
National Bureau of Economic Research

Michael Schlessinger, M.D.
Professor, H. Humphrey Center for Experimental Medicine and
Cancer Research, Jerusalem, Israel

Anne Scitovsky
Chief, Health Economics Department, Palo Alto Medical Foundation

# AIDS AND ECONOMICS:  AN INTERNATIONAL PERSPECTIVE

Daniel Fox, Ph.D.[1]
J. B. Brunet, M.D.[2], and
Rashi Fein, Ph.D.[3]

## INTRODUCTION

### Dr. Fox

Our speakers and panelists this morning will talk about economics.  A subject which is invariably, it seems, addressed at the end of most conferences about AIDS.

Veteran members of panels on AIDS and Economics are familiar with the thinned audiences that dutifully await our remarks on the costs, both direct and indirect, of treating persons with AIDS, on the problems of paying the costs for AIDS patients in countries which lack national health insurance, and on the special burden of AIDS on the scarce resources of developing countries.  As you will soon hear, AIDS raises these issues, but it also raises others of great importance.

Moreover, as you will hear, just as war and medicine are too important to be entrusted to generals and doctors, the economics of epidemic disease must be addressed beyond the community of professional economists.  Our speakers this morning will be addressing three things that have been central to the productive relationship between medicine and the social sciences during the past quarter century.  I will state these themes abstractly.  Our speakers and panelists will provide many practical examples of them.

The first theme is the inseparability of social science, economics in particular, and epidemiology.  The incidence and prevalence of disease can only be discussed intelligently in the context of economic and social history and of the analysis of the way societies currently organize themselves.  The AIDS epidemic, for instance, cannot be understood without studying the movement of workers and tourists and the international flow of blood and blood products.

[1]  Director, New York State Center for Assessing Health Services, State University of New York at Stony Brook  [2]  Director, World Health Organization Collaborating Center on AIDS, Paris, France  [3]  Professor, Economics of Medicine, Harvard Medical School

The second theme is the reliance of medicine on social science to describe and evaluate its interventions and in particular to assess public health practice. In regard to AIDS there is great debate about the relative merits of what those of us in the field of health services research call regulatory and marketing models of intervention. In regulatory models, public authorities set rules and penalize people who do not obey them. In market models, people are educated, given incentives to engage in particular behaviors.

The third theme is the most familiar: The role of social scientists and economists in particular in describing how societies allocate scarce resource and prescribing how resources could be allocated more effectively.

This morning you will hear both description and prescription. Three of our speakers and panelists will describe how people in different countries have addressed problems of allocating resources. Others will tell you how both national wealth and the structure of particular health systems drive the allocation of resources. And one of them will present the results of careful studies of relative costs of treating AIDS and other diseases in the United States. Several of our speakers and panelists will also prescribe as well and describe. They will tell you what they believe ought to be done as a result of both scientific analysis and sound values.


DISCUSSION


Dr. Brunet

It has been said several times that AIDS is now a worldwide problem. To what extent is it really a worldwide problem, what are the situations that different countries have to cope with, what are the possibilities, the strategies against this disease? These are the main points that I will try to develop.

At the end of May 1986, 92 countries have reported their situation to the World Health Organization in Geneva. About a third of these countries have reported no cases, and the total number of cases reported now in the world is about 25,000.

About 80 percent of these cases have been reported from the United States. The State of New York accounts for nearly 30 percent of the total number of cases reported in the world.

What do these figures mean? They provide good estimates of the situation in some countries, and are irrelevant in others. The surveillance of AIDS is not very well conducted in all countries, particularly in the regions of the world in which the disease seems to be the most aggressive.

What is happening in the Americas? Small countries in the Caribbean areas seem to have the highest incidence in the world - higher than that in the United States (rates per million inhabitants: Bermuda: 493; Bahamas: 190; USA: 89). But obviously it is not possible to compare a small island with a small population with a large country with over 2 million inhabitants. But if the situation in the small islands is compared with that in the main towns which are now afflicted with AIDS in the United States it can be seen that the problem seems to be similar in both cases.

Within the American region two countries, Canada and Brazil, seem to be faced with AIDS in the same manner as the European region. It is interesting to note that the 377 cases from Haiti were reported·to WHO by June 1985. Since then no new cases have been reported from Haiti.

The situation in Japan is quite interesting. Only 14 cases have been recorded in Japan (population over 130 million inhabitants). This is not because the surveillance system is not good; in fact, the surveillance system in Japan is as good as in any developed country and there have been some very active efforts to find AIDS cases in Japan. Among the 14 cases reported, half of them are hemophiliac patients treated with imported products from the United States. The first case of AIDS in a homosexual man in Japan was recorded in a Japanese artist who used to live in the U.S.A.

The situation in Africa is less clear than anywhere else in the world. Now 9 African countries have reported their situation to WHO. Of these, 3 countries have reported no cases.

However, countries in which the most extensive studies are now conducted, like Zaire or Rwanda, have not officially reported any cases of AIDS; so we are unable to describe the real situation in Africa. Six countries (Central African Republic, Kenya, South Africa, Tanzania, Tunisia and Uganda) reported a total of 378 cases by the end of May 1986. The fact that these countries have reported cases is very important because this is the first sign that the problem has been recognized in Africa. Perhaps, following these first countries, the other countries in Central Africa will recognize the problem and begin to struggle against this new disease.

Europe is quite particular because, as far as I know, it is the only region in the world which has developed a common surveillance system for AIDS. Now 26 European countries are very kindly collaborating, providing our Centre every quarter with their surveillance data.

Of these 26 countries, 3 (France, United Kingdom, Federal Republic of Germany) account for over 60 percent of all the recorded cases. Cases in eastern Europe were reported not very long ago by Czechoslovakia, which reported 4 cases at March 1986. Yugoslavia reported its first case in September 1985, and now has three cases. In other east European countries which report to our Centre, no cases have been officially reported; but the USSR Ministry of Health reported several cases a few weeks ago at a WHO meeting in Geneva.

The epidemic trend in Europe seems to be similar to that in the USA, but the number of cases is of course much less: 2,500 reported cases in 26 European countries. The same kind of epidemic trend is occurring in nearly every European country.

The European countries most affected seem to be Switzerland and Denmark, which, although small numbers of cases have been reported, have a higher rate per million population (17 and 16 cases per million population respectively).

The situation in Belgium is quite particular among the European countries since about 70 percent of the cases have been reported among African immigrants.

The comparison of the situation in Europe and the United States show some notable differences.

The homosexual group of patients (homosexual and bisexual men) accounts for almost 70 percent of the patients in both the USA and Europe. There is also a similarity in the proportion of transfusion recipients which accounts for 2 percent in both areas.

However the other groups show some differences.

Hemophiliac cases account for 1 percent of the total number of cases reported in the USA, and 4 percent of the European cases. The difference is very probably linked to the fact that the AIDS epidemic in the hemophiliac group began at the same time in Europe and in the USA since most European countries import their blood products from the USA.

The second difference is in the IV drug addicts which accounts for 17 percent of the patients in the United States and only 10 percent in Europe. One year ago only 2% of European AIDS cases were IV drug abusers. This is probably the group in which the disease has spread the fastest in the European countries. I do not think this difference will remain since the proportion of drug abusers among European cases will certainly increase.

The third difference is in the group of patients recorded as having no known risk factor. The proportion of this group in the USA is about 7 percent and in Europe about 15 percent. This difference is due to the large proportion of patients who are African immigrants recorded in Europe. If patients of European origin only are considered, the situation is very similar to that in the USA, and the percentage of patients recorded as having no known risk factor is about 7 percent.

What does this mean? The idea of patients with no known risk factor has been very confusing. In fact, not belonging to an identified risk group does not mean that the mode of transmission of the disease is unknown. Patients from Africa are generally young males and females who have acquired the disease by the same mode of transmission as the European or US patients: by sexual transmission or by infected injection materials.

Particularities of the AIDS epidemic in Africa has led to questionable hypotheses on modes of transmission. Unwise speculation has caused a lot of harm to African countries, not only because of its impact on tourism, but also because it has contributed to delay the awareness of the real problem.

The situation must, however, be considered to be very serious in Africa and some studies which have been conducted in a careful way have shown clearly that the prevalence of the infection in the general population in countries in central Africa is very high, much higher than the prevalence in developed countries so far. For example, one of the studies has looked at the prevalence of HIV in young mothers and found that 5 percent of them were HIV positive in 1980. The AIDS epidemic in Africa affects simultaneously two generations. The fact that a large proportion of young women of child-bearing age in central Africa are infected with the virus is probably one of the main problems with which these countries will have to cope.

Serological studies are also extremely useful for evaluating the situation in countries in which no clinical AIDS cases have been recorded yet. In Hungary, which has not recorded any cases of AIDS so far, testing male homosexuals showed that 5 percent were infected. This seems to be comparable to the situation in San Francisco at the end of the 70's before the first AIDS cases were recognized. This means that even if the AIDS epidemic is not apparent in a country, such as Hungary, the virus may already be present. It also indicates clearly that in such countries it is necessary to try and implement the strategies which are necessary to prevent the epidemic.

The prevalence of seropositive subjects among Hungarian hemophiliacs is about 33 percent among those who have been treated with imported concentrates, and 0 percent for those who have been treated with exclusively domestic products. This situation can be found in several countries in the world which import blood products. Another study conducted in Yugoslavia was also reported by the Yugoslavian Ministry of Health at a WHO European meeting in Graz (Austria). Whereas none of 22,000 blood donors was found to be seropositive, 2.5% (6 out of 239) of the male homosexuals tested, and 33% (165 out of 496) of the drug addicts had anti-HIV antibodies. The spread of the virus among European drug addicts is one of the characteristics of the situation in the southern part of our continent.

In Italy and Switzerland the increase of the prevalence of HIV antibodies has been extremely rapid: 6 percent in 1980 to 76 percent in 1985 in Italy, and from 16 percent in 1982 to 37 percent in 1985 in Switzerland. The recent reports in the United Kingdom are quite surprising for two reasons. First, because the increase seems to be very low: 1.5 percent in 1983 to only 6 percent in 1985; secondly because other authors have reported a very high prevalence of HIV antibodies among drug abusers (as much as 60 percent) in the Scottish region.

Facing the AIDS problem, what are the various public health approaches? The most common response in most countries is screening blood donations. At the end of 1985, 16 European countries have already undertaken programs to screen all blood donors. Since then, other countries, particularly in the eastern countries, have also begun to screen their blood donors. But this kind of response is very limited since transfusion recipients only account for a very low percentage of the AIDS cases.

So what can be done apart from testing the blood donors? It seems that two kinds of strategies have been developed.

The first one is a modern approach in the history of the infectious disease. It is based on the responsibility of the risk groups and their capacity to act as a community faced with a common problem. But this type of approach only works if a community exists which is not the case everywhere or for every risk group. The term "Gay Community" probably has a meaning here in New York and San Francisco, and probably also for a few thousands of people in the main capital cities of Europe. But it is less clear in the rest of the world.

Health education programs are based on a similar approach. Aimed at the general public they have to face many difficulties. Talking openly about sexual practices is not very common for health authorities, even in our so-called "advanced societies." At an individual level, changing sexual behaviour probably requires a very strong motivation. How to develop this in the general public, providing realistic knowledge of what is dangerous, and what is not, without creating panic reactions? That is one of the numerous challenges we have to face.

The second approach is a classical one, with a long historical background in the field of infectious diseases. It is not based on the responsibility of the risk groups but on repression. It involves strategies like contact tracing with more or less confidentiality. It could involve quarantine and restriction of immigration. This kind of approach is considered in some countries, and felt unacceptable in others. The choice of approach is probably more related to the general attitude of the society towards minorities rather than to an assessment of cost efficiency.

In conclusion we can say that the AIDS phenomenon shows three pictures. Several countries are in a pre-epidemic situation: various degrees of this situation are found in West and North Africa, in eastern Europe, the Middle East, in Asia and in most parts of the Pacific region. This situation is characterized by the absence of AIDS cases or very few known AIDS cases, evidence of a low prevalence of infection in high risk groups, a low level of public interest compared to that observed in developed countries.

The second situation is the epidemic situation observed in developed countries. There, the majority of cases have been recorded in high risk groups in which a high prevalence of HIV infection is registered. In contrast, there is a low prevalence of infection in the general population. There are specific public health programs that have been implemented and also a high public interest.

The third group in which there is also an epidemic situation includes countries from central Africa and some countries from the Carribean area which have to cope with the most difficult situation. Most difficult because there are not clearly identified risk groups except prostitutes; because there is a high prevalence of HIV infection in the general population; but also because the health resources are very poor. Although there is a high public interest, no specific health programs have yet been implemented. This is why it is of absolute importance, if we want to cope with AIDS on a worldwide basis, to consider the problem in these countries and to try and help them face the situation. It is obvious that they cannot manage with their own resources. Thank you very much.


## Dr. Fein

What I would like to do in this paper is focus on the similarities between AIDS and other conditions, between the way the health system deals with AIDS and its effects and the way it deals with other health issues, and between the way we think about AIDS and the way we consider other aspects of health care policy. I want to examine those matters, particularly in relation to the economic dimensions of the disease and the economic issues raised.

I stress this similarity for two reasons. First, because I believe we can gain insight into a new problem, AIDS, by looking for and considering aspects of the existing health system and how it handles diseases which are older and with which we are more familiar. The health sector which the individual with AIDS encounters is part of and a reflection of a wider health sector and its organization and priorities. We will gain insights on something new by considering its relationship to older terrain over which we have traveled.

The second reason for considering potential similarities is equally important. How public and private policy is shaped in relation to AIDS may tell us something about policies that may be pursued for good and for bad in other arenas. Policies developed to respond to AIDS may become more generalized in the future. And in that very important sense some of the issues in AIDS policy become issues that stretch beyond AIDS and are necessarily issues in health care policy in its broadest dimension.

I stress, of course, that the attempt to tease out or discuss some of the similarities between AIDS and other conditions is not meant to minimize AIDS' special significance. If we list all of AIDS' characteristics and implications, we cannot dispute that it is unique. And still I do believe that we can gain the insight and understanding by examining the various individual characteristics and our experience with other conditions that exhibit one or more of those characteristics. Thus we may learn something about the economics of AIDS by considering general issues in health care organization and financing and at the same time we may learn something about those general issues by considering how we attempt to deal with AIDS.

AIDS forces us to think about the limitations and misallocations of the existing medical care delivery and financing system. It does so because the issues it raises are too large to be conveniently ignored and because its very novelty and the way it has burst upon the scene has dramatized its impact. For a variety of reasons with which all of us are familiar, AIDS calls for explicit policy decisions and many of those decisions force us to confront existing inadequacies in the organization of health services and in their financing.

Similarly we are forced to recognize the areas of intersection and overlap between health care policy and social policy, a set of issues that arises elsewhere in medical care but one which is often ignored though not without real cost.

Let me begin by noting some of the characteristics that AIDS shares with other conditions. Much of the treatment for AIDS involves long term ambulatory care requiring effective followup and counseling. Over a significant period of time, the resources required by those with AIDS as well as by those who do not manifest AIDS symptoms but have tested positive for the antibody are the very resources that our medical care system seems to have in short supply.

I refer, of course, to the skills of counselors, nurses and social workers and the ability to organize, mobilize and manage multiple sources of care and assistance. The U.S. medical care system's orientation to acute care and, to a significant degree, to hospital based services, is at variance with the needs in chronic care, and much of AIDS treatment has characteristics akin to chronic care.

The reasons for our shortfall and the provision in our handling of chronic care are many. First, there is a reliance on a science based medical model that is often interpreted incorrectly, but nonetheless as if it calls for a choice between science and competence on the one hand and humanity and warmth on the other.

Furthermore, there is a status and hierarchy legacy reflected in and supported by the fact that most physicians commonly called curers were and are male, and most nurses, counselors and social workers often called carers were and are female. In addition, the difficulty of organization of diverse services by multiple providers to ambulatory patients who are not conveniently available in a hospital bed is a factor. The bias is toward hospital-based medical education and toward a financing system which historically has driven the care system toward in-hospital services.

AIDS, therefore, calls on the health sector to organize itself and to provide the very services it has historically undervalued. Perhaps this is one time that the health sector will respond adequately, but we cannot underrate the obstacles - which is to say that the right things won't happen by themselves. They require public policy interventions that reverse historical trends and priorities.

As we all know, AIDS does require acute and in-hospital services. Many patients die while they are receiving those services. Thus, as with other persons, expenditures mount rapidly at the end of life. Since patterns of care, especially as between in and out of hospital services vary widely across the nation, and since as yet we are not certain of the length of the latency period and therefore at what point in time to begin to count the costs of AIDS treatment, it is impossible to estimate what percentage of the total expenditures on AIDS comes in the last six months or last year of life.

Nevertheless, it is clear that the percentage, as with many other conditions and with other population groups, for example, the very aged, is high. Dramatic as these data may be, we must guard against drawing false inferences for public policy. If the data tell us anything, they tell us to search for alternative modalities of care, though we cannot assume that we will always find them, and in any case, we ought not to need dramatic data to encourage us to search for alternatives. The data do not tell us, although that appears what some persons read into them, that high expenditures near the end of life are a waste of resources - for the aged, for burn victims, for individuals with AIDS.

The health sector, after all, does not have only one goal - one output measure - the avoidance of death. It has numerous goals, and among them, the easing of pain and suffering. The fact that resources are allocated to AIDS and other patients who are terminally ill reflects a value structure and orientation that few of us would deplore. It is possible that that orientation will change, but surely there can be no double standard that calls for different policies for terminally ill patients - depending on the disease with which they are afflicted.

AIDS shares yet another characteristic with other conditions. How we deal with the disease, both in terms of the resources allocated to it, and in the way that these costs are shared, is heavily influenced by attitudes toward those who contract it, and to the degree that we can attribute its presence through lifestyle and behavior - and as we've learned from various questions during this conference - especially, of course, behavior that is "morally wrong". I do not, of course, imply that AIDS and those that contract it are viewed in precisely the same way as those who drink, smoke or eat too much, drive too fast or exercise too little. I do suggest, however, that in the United States, the recent emphasis on the individual's personal role in disease prevention and health promotion coupled with the suggestion that one hears that the right to health care should be coupled with the responsibility to promote one's own health - provides a presumed intellectual rationale for existing biases.

I surely need not point out that this is particularly the case with AIDS - a disease in which the principal high risk groups - homosexual males and IV drug abusers - are especially stigmatized. And yet, though AIDS is different, it is part of a regrettable attitude - an old attitude in the social arena and a new one in health affairs - that of blaming the victim.

These and other similarities between the various ramifications of AIDS and other health conditions suggest that AIDS dramatically highlights the problem of allocation of resources within the U.S. health care system. It does so because AIDS stresses the health care system precisely in those places where it is already under stress.

I shall not spell out but invite each of you to consider the problems faced by AIDS patients and those close to them as they encounter the health care system and the problems faced by Alzheimer patients - the similarities are apparent.

One point of stress involves the financing of care, and it is to that important issue that I would now direct our attention. Up to this point, it is perhaps the case that the problems faced by individuals with AIDS in the United States are not too dissimilar from those faced by patients in many other industrial nations, since the skewing of the health delivery system to acute rather than chronic care, to in-hospital rather than out-of-hospital services, and the failure to integrate social and medical services and the consequent substitution of more expensive medical services for more effective social services is not a uniquely U.S. phenomenon. But when we turn to financing of care, the contrast between the United States and other industrial nations is sharp indeed. The United States does have systems of insurance - some private and some public - but has approached the provision of insurance by focusing on beneficiary groups defined by various socio-economic or demographic characteristics such as age, employment, income, disease - rather than focusing on universality.

Where other nations define the benefits that are available, we define the beneficiaries who will be served. Nor do we operate within a health budget or something that approximates a set of decisions taken about the level of expenditures for care. Our expenditures are only known ex post and are the outcome of billions of largely private decisions.

The financial implication of AIDS on patients, institutions and the public purse, are great. But different parts of the financing system fund different parts of the expenditures and therefore have been affected in different ways. Let me examine some of those ways. I begin by directing our attention at the financing problem faced by AIDS patients and those who have tested positive for the antibody and who are therefore at higher risk of becoming individuals with AIDS. The first group - those with AIDS - is not a very large group in terms of absolute numbers. At present levels, total expenditures even at the high cost estimated by CDC - and we'll hear more about that later - would not represent a cost that would strain the U.S. economy or even the U.S. health sector were those costs spread over the total economy or total health sector total society.

In his President's letter, Bruce Vladeck, President of the United Hospital Fund of New York notes that even at CDC estimates, hospital spending for AIDS is only 3/10 of one percent of the nation's health bill. If we presume that economic pressure either catalyzes or forces reallocations that induce the search for more efficiency, I believe it is perhaps fair to say that expenditures on AIDS are not generally so large as to result in an active search for and development of new modalities of care.

I do not suggest, of course, that the economic spur is the only thing that would lead us to look for new modalities of care, since examples of other ways of dealing with the problem do exist, and since health workers and persons with AIDS are interested, vitally interested in this, there's going to be that search. But I do suggest it's not going to be spurred in many communities by the economic pressure. Of course, however, this is only the case generally. We recognize that some communities are especially affected. The average figure is not particularly reassuring to those cities any more so than a person drowning in the Mississippi finds solace and comfort in the statement that the average depth of the river is only 2 inches.

Furthermore, the number of AIDS patients is increasing and for reasons that we shall come to, the pressure on public funds for health care may increase even more sharply. Over time, an increasing number of communities will question the existing patterns of in-hospital care and in the longer run, we are therefore likely to find that the increase in the number of patients will be associated with new and different treatment modalities and with reductions in per patient expenditures.

Whether the arithmetic product of these two variables - the number of individuals times the cost per individual - will increase or decrease is unclear. I am not arguing that total expenditures will decline or even that they will stabilize. All that I am suggesting, in the current atmosphere of panic about explosive expenditures is that (1) we don't have enough information to estimate future cost implications; (2) there is reason to believe on the basis of our experience with AIDS and our more general knowledge about health care services that care can be produced in many different ways with many different combinations of inputs and at many different levels of expenditures; (3) rapidly rising costs are likely in this as in other areas of economic activity to lead to changes in behavior (in this case, treatment) to a search for alternatives and to new combinations of input, and (4) therefore that extrapolations of present cost per patient into the future -

even a future in which there are many more patients - will lead to gross overestimates of future expenditures.

It is irresponsible to suggest that America will not be able to afford to treat those with AIDS. It is irresponsible on two counts -- one to the economists "to be able to afford" really is the wrong phrase since it means do you choose to treat, do you choose to spend, -- but in this case, I would suggest for the four reasons cited, that it is also irresponsible.

Nevertheless, in the short run, the panic attitude is not likely to be entirely dispelled. And if that indeed is the case, we are likely to find groups trying to shift what they see as potentially high costs onto someone else's budget. It is therefore not surprising, though I do find it shocking, that we witness attempts to segment the insurance markets, attempts by those who have insurance and don't believe that they will come in contact with the virus, to disassociate themselves from those who they believe are at greater risk - attempts by insurers who want to compete through lower premiums to make certain that they don't cover high cost subscribers, and attempts by employers who don't want to buy insurance for people who will turn out to be expensive, to make certain that those people don't enter their group of subscribers.

At an earlier stage of our development of voluntary health insurance when community rated premiums were the prevailing pattern, the incentive to define individuals out of one's group was less, though the incentive, of course, to define them out of insurance in general, would still have been present, albeit in attenuated form.

Today, when experience rating and self-insurance by employers dominate, the incentive to exclude those who are likely to need costly care is greater. Furthermore, given the increase in concern about rising health care costs over the last decade, the increase of efforts to control costs at the firm and plant level in contrast to more general approaches directed at system behavior or price controls, the increased attention to costs containment by reductions in utilization, the increased health sector competition with its increased emphasis on price differentials - and I believe the increased awareness by insurers of the cost of insurance - the incentives to define some people out of the insurance sector will continue to grow.

The private insurance sector, employers, employees, HMOs and other delivery systems still to be invented, will all try to shift potential cost elsewhere.

Where are and who are those elsewheres? It should be obvious that cost cannot be shifted readily to AIDS patients. These persons are not generally characterized by high incomes and large savings accounts. Nor are they able to purchase individual insurance on their own and even if they had group insurance while employed, many of them are likely to have lost it as a consequence of their illness and withdrawal from the labor force. Thus, the attempt to shift costs to the public sector. Medicare for the disabled can begin the 30th month after the first full calendar month of disability - hardly much of a help. Medicaid via the medically needy program may be available, but without a federal contribution and only in some states. Pools to deal with uncompensated care may be available, but again, only in some states - largely for hospital care and in-hospital care. As elsewhere in health financing the patterns of payment provide incentives for in-rather than out-of-hospital treatment.

While patterns will vary across the country in many places, therefore, it is local government that is most at risk by city or county support for a public hospital. It can be argued that public support for AIDS treatment expenditures is or could be more equitable than private funding through health insurance premiums which are unrelated after all to income and ability to pay.

Many of those who have supported national health insurance in the United States have argued just that point. Clearly, however, when they made that argument, they did not envision that the term public support excluded the federal government, excluded much of state government and was therefore to be defined as a disproportionate use of city tax revenues. In general, the situation faced by our major cities is not yet severe. Nevertheless, it is likely to grow severe as a consequence in the number of AIDS patients and decreases in federal support for their general budgets and for specific programs that cities value and will want to retain. Some cities do have a disproportionate share of AIDS patients. Surely that calls for a system of cost sharing that broadens rather than narrows the net through which the dollars might flow. I note that Fred Robbins referred to universal health insurance; I note that Harvey Feinberg referred to a new system of pooling arrangements, and I think that it's high time for a group of individuals to sit down, put their ideas together and try and work out within the American tradition, focusing on beneficiary groups, a feasible and sensible program for the financing in this arena. That would not deny anybody the right and privilege to continue to fight for universal health insurance, but it would suggest, I suppose, that to postpone doing something in this area in order to advance universal health insurance is somewhat irresponsible.

I believe that there are things in this arena that can be done. The argument for a wider sharing of costs is, I believe, made even more compelling if one recognizes that those communities that develop and organize better treatment patterns and that fund these through the public sector and philanthropy are likely to attract yet more persons in need of care, thus creating yet more stress in an already stressful situation.

The problems created by migration patterns of AIDS patients are likely to be made even more compelling if we take into account the possible behavior of the much larger population of individuals who have tested positive for the antibody and of those not tested but who are aware that their behavior puts them at high risk. Given their knowledge that in some communities they will fare better than in others, given the latency period which provides time for migration, we could expect additional inflow of potential AIDS patients.

Since, in addition, those communities that are organized to deliver better care are likely to be found in states that discourage or bar mandatory testing by insurers and employers, the incentive for in-migration is further increased. It is, I believe, evident that in a world in which the issues raised by AIDS are dealt with in a fragmented way by individual cities and states it will become increasingly costly and difficult for states with open borders to continue to behave in what they view as a more enlightened fashion than their neighbors. It is tough to be a good guy in a bad world.

I believe that in this area, as in others already mentioned, the similarity between the way society reacts to AIDS and the way it deals or will choose to deal with other conditions is striking.

Just last week, one of our TV stations in Boston carried a discussion of the new testing procedures that may enable us to determine the risk that an individual faces of contracting any one of a number of diseases. One of the points made in that story was repeated in USA Today just yesterday that the result of such tests could be used by employers and by health insurers presumably to disengage from high risk employees and subscribers.

And thus, I suggest that if, with AIDS - why not with hypertension. And if with hypertension - why not with AIDS. Recent and continuing improvements and advances in testing and screening enable us to assess individual risks more accurately than in the past. While none of us would dispute the many benefits that screening may confer, we should recognize and discuss the problems it raises. We are required - and not simply in the case of AIDS - to ask what purpose a particular screening or testing program would serve - what actions would one take in response to results - who would derive the benefits - who would have access to the data. Improved technology requires that these kinds of questions be asked and answered. In the last few years, our health care delivery and financing system has embraced the reality of competition. To be sure, competition has many positive aspects, but it has negative consequences as well.

We should be aware that insurers and deliverers of care may choose to compete for low risk populations rather than around efficiency considerations. It is simply the case that more money called profits or excess of operating revenues over expenditures in the non-profit sector, can be made by making certain that one is not responsible for treating or paying for patients who are likely to be expensive.

If screening can predict who those patients are, if we permit and encourage segmentation of the population, we will destroy our health financing system and abandon those who most need help.

How we react, in other words, how we react to the individual with AIDS - thus offers a dramatic insight to a more general health care financing problem which I fear we will encounter more frequently in the future. What the future holds for AIDS financing is not unrelated to our more general financing of care and to the strains and stresses that we will place on that system and as a consequence, on our public hospitals already under stress. We are likely to lose our sense of community and I would suggest that for selfish reasons, if for no other reasons, persons without AIDS and persons who are convinced that they will never be infected, ought to be concerned because everyone is, in some sense, viewed by others as a member of some minority group.

I am not here to issue a report card on the health care system's response to AIDS. It's kind of a meaningless question in the United States. San Francisco is not Phoenix, Boston is not Peoria, etc. What I would suggest is that if the grade that each of us might give is not as high as we believe it should be or we would like we not hide behind the excuse that AIDS came upon us suddenly and that we simply haven't had time to adjust to its impact.

Of course, AIDS is a new phenomenon. But if we are dealing
inadequately with its impact on the delivery and financing of care,
it is in no small measure because we generally deal inadequately
with those issues. AIDS, therefore, can serve to highlight those
inadequacies and can serve to remind us of the need to solve those
more general problems. Perhaps in highlighting these problems, AIDS
will encourage us to solve them to the benefit not only of AIDS
patients, but of our entire society.

Thank you.


COMMENTS


Fakhry Assaad, M.D., M.P.H. (Director, Division of Communicable
Diseases, World Health Organization, Geneva, Switzerland)

There is no doubt that AIDS and ARC are costly diseases in human
as well as financial terms. Due to the predominantly sexual mode of
transmission, over 90 percent of cases in the developing world - as
in the developed world - are in the age groups 20 to 49 years of
age. This is the most productive age. Thus, the loss of human
potential has to also be added to the financial burden. Dr. Fein
mentioned medical ethics. However, for a poor country, one has to
recognize that taking care of AIDS patients is not an investment in
health. It is just taking care of patients, and this, for a poor
country certainly poses a heavy burden on health services. Dr.
Brunet mentioned the three categories of countries. I will
concentrate on the third group of countries, many of which are
characterized epidemiologically by heterosexual transmission as well
as transmission by nonsterile needles and syringes and other skin-
or mucous membrane-piercing instruments. These countries have a
high number of prenatal and pediatric cases. They also have
apparent transmission through uncontrolled and unscreened blood
transfusions. As Dr. Brunet said, these countries also face the
impact of other diseases, such as measles, malaria, within a context
of malnutrition as well. In Africa it is estimated that between one
and two million or even more persons are infected with HIV virus.
If we conservatively consider only one million infected, and we
consider the most conservative rate of annual progression to AIDS -
that is one percent - we can estimate a minimum of 10,000 AIDS cases
occurring in Africa per year. This represents a bleak picture of
what we have to face in the African situation. To confront the
problem of HIV infection, we have established the WHO Programme on
AIDS. We have invested, thus far, over a million dollars of very
scarce international resources. WHO believes that AIDS is indeed an
exceptional public health problem which represents a global health
challenge.

The WHO program has been very well received by the governing
bodies of WHO. The World Health Assembly, the supreme governing
body of the World Health Organization representing 166 countries,
recently requested the Director-General to act in response to the
AIDS challenge and endorsed WHO's role as a coordinator for

multilateral as well as bilateral control and research efforts.

The support of national efforts for the control of AIDS is the most important component of the WHO program. The prerequisite step in this collaborative effort would have to be an indication on the part of a Member State of national willingness to confront the complex problem associated with HIV infections. A comprehensive plan at the national level begins with a political commitment through the establishment of a national AIDS committee formed and coordinated by the Ministry of Health and including appropriate representatives of other relevant ministries as well.

The lack of health infrastructures at the country level that can effectively address the AIDS problem represents the major obstacle we face in the developing world. Therefore, the design of a national program requires the initial assessment of the problem. This initial assessment has two components: The epidemiological assessment to determine the prevalence of HIV in selected areas; and the resource infrastructure assessment to determine the ability of existing health systems to support epidemiological, laboratory, clinical and preventive components of a national program.

Based on these findings, a surveillance system has to be implemented, a difficult task in a country with limited infrastructure, capabilities and funds. In addition, laboratory support is required. Can we create reference laboratories on a global scale? How many? Can we establish intercountry collaboration, cooperation, coordination - to provide laboratory services for more than one country in any one area, for instance? National health programs have to be assisted in the recognition, diagnosis and management of AIDS cases.

The principal goal of any control program directed toward AIDS, however, is prevention. And here again we rely on education and public health communication strategies. If one considers the many languages that may exist in any one country, the existing literacy rate, and varying customs and beliefs, educational strategies will have to be appropriately geared to these populations in any one country.

We will soon be convening a group of experts in public health communication in June. Their role will be to advise us on how we can help Member States approach this problem in the developing world. We will need some success in this area if we are to stem the increasing transmission potential of this virus.

To initiate AIDS prevention and control efforts in a country of approximately 10 million in Africa, we will need close to half a million U.S. dollars. This represents the cost involved in initiating the program, however, and is not a sufficient amount for maintaining the program over time. We do not expect that any country affected by adverse economic conditions can contribute more than 20 percent of the cost. We will therefore need an average of 400,000 U.S. dollars from extrabudgetary sources for each country with a population of about 10 million. We have calculated that we need approximately 13 million U.S. dollars to implement the necessary collaborative activities during the 1986-87 biennium.

The situations in a number of countries are critical. We cannot wait any longer. AIDS and HIV infection have already spread far beyond acceptable boundaries.

The United States delegation to the World Health Assembly has stated that it would be contributing $2,000,000 to WHO in support of this program. At the end of next month, we will convene a meeting of potential donor and potential recipient countries. We hope we will be successful in our extrabudgetary fund-raising activities.

The WHO global program itself has six components which comprise the following: exchange of information, preparation and distribution of guidelines, assessment of diagnostic methodology for HIV infection; cooperation with Member States; advice to Member States on the provision of safe blood and blood products; and coordination of research.

From WHO headquarters, we would like to fund two pilot programs so that in collaborating with the respective Governments, we can learn more about prevention and control strategies, thus helping us to more effectively collaborate with other countries. WHO believes that AIDS represents a unique public health problem and indeed a global challenge for national, bilateral and multilateral agencies.


Anne Scitovsky (Chief, Health Economics Department, Palo Alto Medical Foundation)

I want to discuss very briefly two studies we've conducted on the economic costs of the AIDS epidemic in the United States. The first is a retrospective study of the cost of treatment of all AIDS patients treated at San Francisco General Hospital in 1984. As you have heard yesterday, San Francisco General Hospital in 1984 treated about half of all AIDS patients in San Francisco, or about 5 percent of all AIDS patients in the United States.

The second study consists of estimates of the direct and indirect costs of the AIDS epidemic in the United States in 1985, 1986 and 1990. This latter study was conducted at the request of the Centers for Disease Control (CDC), who supplied us with estimates of the prevalence of AIDS in those three years.

Let me go very briefly over the first study. It generated three sets of data. The first set consists of data on average costs per admission by diagnosis. We grouped diagnoses into six categories: Pneumocystis carinii pneumonia (PCP), Kaposi's sarcoma, other infectious diseases, diseases of the blood, diseases of the nervous system and all others lumped together.

The second set of data consists of average expenditures of AIDS patients who received all their in-patient and out-patient care at San Francisco General Hospital in 1984. Excluded were non-institutional expenses like nursing home care, home health care, counseling and similar expenses, so it's only services they received as in-patients and out-patients at San Francisco General.

The final data consists of the lifetime hospital costs of AIDS patients who died in 1984 and had received all their in-patient care at San Francisco General Hospital.

I won't discuss the first two data. The most interesting, I think, are the data on lifetime costs. We found the lifetime hospital costs at San Francisco General Hospital of patients who died came to just under $30,000. This is very much lower than the very high estimate of $147,000 that was made by Dr. Anne Hardy of the Centers for Disease Control in early 1985.

You have all heard that San Francisco is different, so I won't go into all the differences. But by no stretch of the imagination could I arrive at a figure of $147,000. I collected data from all over the country on average length of stay, average number of hospitalizations over a lifetime of the patient, and on average charges per hospital day for the Centers of Disease Control estimate and I would say average lifetime costs of AIDS patients may range somewhere between $50,000 and $100,000, but more likely between $60,000 and $75,000 in 1984 dollars.

Since I made that very rough estimate I have heard similar figures from several other sources.

Let me add just one point to this lifetime costs. What has got lost in the public discussion of the CDC estimate (and I'm emphasizing the CDC estimate, because it has received such wide publicity) is that their figure of $147,000 refers to lifetime costs. As a matter of fact in the article, these lifetime costs are compared with annual costs of other diseases.

The confusion is understandable because the average lifetime of an AIDS patient is not very long - very little more than a year - but it should be borne in mind. Unfortunately we don't have data on the lifetime costs of other diseases, at least I have not been able to find anything reasonably recent. However, I made an estimate based on Medicare data of lifetime costs of end-stage renal disease patients who are on dialysis. As you may know, end-stage renal disease is covered by Medicare which has very good data on annual expenditures per case. I came up with an estimate of lifetime costs of some $158,000 for this particular disease, very much higher than any possible lifetime cost that I can see for AIDS and somewhat higher than the estimate of Anne Hardy of CDC.

The estimate we prepared for the CDC of the direct and indirect costs of the AIDS epidemic was made by me and Dorothy Rice jointly. I estimated the direct personal health care costs. She estimated the direct non-personal health care costs, that is, costs for research, screening, education and miscellaneous other services not assignable directly to a particular patient. She also estimated the indirect costs, which are the value of lost input due to morbidity and premature mortality.

We made a range of three estimates because of the many uncertainties regarding the course of the epidemic and future costs. The lowest is based on San Francisco merely as an example of how low costs could be if conditions prevailing in San Francisco prevailed nationwide. Let me read you the figures for what I consider our best estimates of direct and indirect costs in these years in current dollars.

For 1985 direct personal health care cost of AIDS patients came to about $630 million. The direct non-personal costs for screening, education, etc. came to about $319 million. However, the indirect costs came to $3.9 billion. The indirect costs are so high because the people who die from AIDS are largely young people in their most productive years of life, hence the indirect cost of loss of earnings over their expected lifetime is very high.

For 1986 the figures are $1.1 billion for the direct personal costs, $542 million for the direct non-personal costs, and $7.0 billion for the indirect costs.

While the direct personal medical care costs estimated for 1985 and 1986 are relatively low and represent only about 0.2 percent of estimated national personal health care expenditures in these years, costs in the later years are very much higher because the CDC estimate a steep rise in the incidence and prevalence of the disease. Projecting current trends, they estimate that there will be 145,000 reported cases of AIDS alive at any time during the year. However, they believe that this figure should be increased by 20 percent to adjust for under-reporting of cases, which brings the estimated number of cases in 1991 to 172,800. Using this higher figure, we estimated direct personal medical care costs of AIDS patients at $8.5 billion in current dollars, direct non-personal costs at $2.3 billion, and indirect costs at $55.6 billion. Direct personal medical care costs according to our estimate would represent about 1.4 percent of estimated national personal health care expenditures in 1991. Thus despite the fact that our estimate of medical care costs of AIDS patients is very much lower than the earlier estimate made by the CDC, total medical care costs for AIDS in the early 1990s are likely to be substantial if the epidemic spreads as estimated by the CDC.

In conclusion, I'd like to make two points. Some people have said to me that by stressing the fact that medical care costs per person with AIDS seem to be lower than originally estimated by the CDC, I may hinder efforts to get more money into the battle against AIDS. However, I don't really believe that. I feel that the panic caused by the early high estimate has scared employers and the insurance industry more than is actually justified and may have led at least some of them to consider ways of restricting employment or insurance coverage for high risk groups. By publicizing more realistic estimates of the costs of treatment of AIDS patients I hope to encourage a more dispassionate look at the epidemic.

Second, when we explored data on the direct non-personal costs of AIDS, we found that at least to date, very little has been spent on education of the public about ways of avoiding infection with the AIDS virus. We estimated that in 1985, the amounts spent for education were about 7 percent of total direct non-personal costs and equalled only about 4 percent of the direct personal medical care costs of persons with AIDS. In view of the importance of education that has been stressed by just about every speaker at this conference, this is very meager. Until a vaccine or a cure have been found for AIDS, our best means of combatting the disease is prevention, and this requires a widespread education effort at the local, state and federal level as well as by private organizations. I hope very much that this serious gap in our fight against the epidemic will be filled, the sooner the better.

Thank you very much.

Victor Fuchs, Ph.D. (Professor of Economics, Stanford University, Research Associate, National Bureau of Economic Research)

As you well know, AIDS is a great medical problem and a great social problem. There are many public policy issues surrounding AIDS and many of those public policy issues have an economic aspect. How much should the country be spending on AIDS? What should that money be used for? How much for treatment? How much for prevention? How much for research? And then within each category: What kinds of treatment? Where? How? Prevention? What kinds of prevention? And so on.

These are all allocation decisions that economists encounter in every aspect of society and presumably the economic way of thinking about these things would make some contribution here. The final basic economic question always is, who pays? And this is the one that I would like to concentrate on in the context of insurance.

I take as my jumping off point an Op Ed from the New York Times that appeared this week. This Op Ed supports a bill that has been proposed by Governor Cuomo to ban the use of blood testing by insurance companies in screening applicants for health insurance, life insurance and disability insurance. The Op Ed argues that this is a matter of civil rights and that it will save money for the tax payers.

Now I didn't come 3,000 miles to take a stand against civil rights or to fight for higher taxes, but I will suggest that the arguments for the bill seem problematical in several respects. First, it seems to me to be important to distinguish between health insurance and life insurance, something that the article does not do and I take it that the bill does not do either.

Let's consider health insurance first and let's get certain things out that we can all agree on. The first is that sick people should get care. Second, that the costs of care for AIDS victims is so high it is unreasonable to expect that the sick people themselves can bear that cost. And third, that the method of funding will not affect the need for care. We are not dealing with a situation here of the kind of moral hazard that some health economists like to talk about.

So what we are really dealing with - if we can agree on all those things - is simply a question of who should pay for the care. That's the issue. I take it that the thrust of the bill, and the Op Ed supporting it is that the payment mechanism should be through conventional insurance mechanisms of one kind or another, primarily as a device to save the taxpayers money. One might ask first of all, does it save any money? No, it doesn't save any money. The costs of taking care of people with AIDS is going to be the same. It simply redistributes who is going to pay for it.

Is that redistribution desirable? Is it a fair distribution? Is it going to be more fairly shared? Is it going to be a more efficient way to fund the costs? I think there's considerable reason to doubt that. Anybody at all familiar with health insurance knows that the costs of health insurance are passed to the buyers of health insurance - the people who buy the insurance, the policy holders, the other people. If it's the employer, it is passed on in wages foregone or higher prices to consumers.

I don't think the cost will be spread fairly. I think it will tend to get concentrated in some occupations and industries, and some health insurance plans will wind up paying much more than others. At a time when the whole thrust of the insurance field is toward experience rating, to fragmentation, to skimming and creaming it seems to me that this will introduce still another element which will distort and in a sense pervert and corrupt the whole idea of private health insurance by relying on that mechanism rather than saying as some of my colleagues have already said, AIDS is a national disaster, and it should be paid for and shared equally by everybody in the country via our tax mechanisms. This is a fairer method and a more efficient method than any other that I can think of.

Life insurance, which I want to distinguish from health insurance, has some similarities but also some differences. It's similar in the sense that the costs of insurance are borne by the people who buy life insurance. That's transparent in the case of mutual insurance companies that account for about half of the industry, buy I assure you that it is equally true of the other kinds of insurance companies, too. There is no Santa Claus out there who can be called upon to bear the costs. People bear those costs.

Where life insurance differs, it seems to me, is in this question of a right, a civil right to life insurance. I don't know quite what that means and I don't know particularly what it means until it's somehow quantified. Is it the right to $10,000 worth of life insurance? $100,000? A million dollars worth of insurance? Life insurance just doesn't seem to be in the same category as talking about sick people who need care.

It has been stated and it is correctly stated that not everyone who tests positively for HIV is necessarily going to get AIDS, and therefore, it's discriminatory to deal with that person in a particular manner. But that's a misrepresentation of the way insurance works. Insurance never works on a basis of certainty. Insurance always works on a basis of probability. Not every cigarette smoker is going to die young. Not every person who is overweight is going to get a heart attack when they are 50 years old and yet the insurance companies attempt to discover who smokes and who is overweight. In fact, insurance companies are being urged to find out who smokes cigarettes and to pursue underwriting policies accordingly.

Thus, one must at least raise some questions about whether this proposed bill actually contributes in any meaningful way to either a more efficient society or to a more equitable or fairer society. I suppose there may be some people at the conference who think that it does and I certainly want to listen to those arguments and hear what they are and try to absorb them. I do appreciate having this opportunity to raise some questions with you and to suggest why the ban on testing advocated by Governor Cuomo and the Op Ed seems problematical.

Michael Schlessinger, M.D. (Professor, H. Humphrey Center for
Experimental Medicine and Cancer Research, Jerusalem, Israel)

Before I address the general topic that we are now discussing,
just a few words about the situation in Israel.  In Israel we have
so far 25 cases of AIDS.  The virus appeared in Israel in October
1979.  This we know, because at that time a certain patient received
an infected transfusion, and later developed the disease.

Of our 25 AIDS patients, five are hemophiliacs and two were
blood transfusion recipients.  Among the 25 are also a number of
aliens or tourists.  The financial situation in Israel is unique in
that first of all our economy is in rather bad shape.  It has
certain problems that are different from other developing
countries.  We have a national debt that is so high that every baby
at birth already has about $7,000 of debt.

The problem of financing health care is a major problem and
there are strains on the system.  Nevertheless, on the positive
side, in health insurance Israel is available to everybody.  Nobody
can be excluded.  This policy has been implemented from the
beginning because Israel is a country for the absorption of
newcomers and, for instance, if we have new immigration from
Ethiopia, nobody asks how many of them have this or that particular
disease and can they be accepted for health insurance.

The health insurance in Israel is implemented by special sick
funds and the vast majority of the population belongs to one of
them.  Part of the finance is carried by the insured individual,
part by the employer, and part by the health ministry - by the
government.  So much about Israel.

I want to address the problems of AIDS policy.  AIDS policy
means actually, in the final analysis, the allocation of funds.  But
we have to examine the commitment that we have to each of the facets
of the fight against AIDS.

We can look at other examples.  For instance, we know how to
prevent car accidents.  Car accidents kill young people in the prime
of life.  Does society do everything it can to prevent it?  Or is
the cost of building new roads, better roads, safer cars, safer
devices too much for society?  How deeply are we involved in this
commitment?

We know that smoking causes cancer.  Now, for instance, in
Israel it is against the law to smoke in a public hall.  But here I
notice that even at a meeting devoted to a medical problem, there
are quite a few smokers around.  I'm really surprised.

So it's not only that we have to know what to do, but we also
have to be fully committed to implement what we know.  In terms of
economy it means that, for instance, as has been said throughout the
meeting, we might need funds for allocation for clean needles for
drug addicts.  But at least we should have a controlled study to
ascertain the feasability of this approach.  Is it good to start a
program to give free needles to drug addicts?  It's high time for
such a study.

We talked here about safe sex.  What does this mean?  Are
condoms the final answer, and if they are, maybe they should be made
available free to the gay community, or to other communities.

161

So we have to define what we mean by AIDS policy and how we are
going to implement it and how much we are going to commit ourselves
in either regulatory or marketing approaches. And, of course, if we
put a lot of effort into education, it's very, very important to
have education repeatedly reinforced and not only just one or two
encounters in ads, but to reinforce it all the time.

As we already said, we have to concentrate our efforts in the
prevention of the disease. The main means for the prevention of the
spread of AIDS will be education, and the testing of blood and blood
products. This may not be an easy task in various countries. In
Israel we had to fight for government approval for the testing of
blood transfusions until quite recently. In Israel all the blood
donated to blood banks began to be screened just six weeks ago.
Initially, this delay was caused by our health ministry, who thought
that the expense of such testing was unjustified in view of the
relatively large proportion of false positive results. After our
health ministry was convinced, our finance ministry thought that the
expense was too high, and we are talking in Israel about a total
expenditure of $1 million. That's 200,000 blood tests at an
estimated cost of $5 each. As a matter of fact, just before I left
Israel to attend this conference, I was informed that two positives
were already identified among blood donors within the first six
weeks of the program.

We have heard and talked a lot about treatment and research in
the field of AIDS. If one reads about the new approaches to AIDS
research one is perplexed by the diametrically conflicting
approaches. Some research groups advocate that one should stimulate
the T-lymphocyte system. This goal could be achieved by the
administration of thymic hormones and by various other
immunomodulators, that would stimulate that system of the immune
mechanism that is most damaged by the disease.

On the other hand we read reports on how important it may be to
do precisely the opposite - to treat AIDS patients with cyclosporin
A, so as to kill the subset of T-lymphocytes that is afflicted by
the disease. On the airplane coming here I read an article
published in the International Herald Tribune in which it was
suggested that AIDS infection of T-cells could be abrogated by
antibodies to thymosine, one of the hormones produced by the thymus.

Before large sums of money are committed to research on the
treatment of AIDS one shouldn't forget that money has to be given
first for pilot studies on how the various methods of treatment
work. One has to avoid a common mistake and remember that our goal
is to treat the disease rather than the symptoms.

Yesterday we heard about a new type of treatment that causes the
HIV virus to disappear, yet the AIDS patients continue to die at the
same rate as untreated patients. We often are attracted to the
administration of new treatments that only alleviate symptoms, but
the patient's fate may not be improved.

What has to come out of this conference, and which is so
important, is that we should be able, each one of us in his
community, in his state, in his environment, to translate the new
insight of the various facets of the disease into commitment, into
the various facets of either education within his circle, or early
diagnosis or modalities of treatment.

The question was raised as to where the funds for the management of AIDS patients should come from? In each country the funds may have to come from different sources. In Israel we expect that the government and the labor sick fund (Kaput Cholim) will carry most of the financial burden.

There may be a need for further funds. The money obtained in various countries from the government at either the national or the municipal level may not be enough for the management of AIDS. It may be necessary to organize voluntary groups as has already been done in San Francisco and in other places, that will supplement the urgent needs, and will also enable the community to participate in deciding how the funds should be distributed. Such voluntary funds may help create in the community a feeling of sharing in a common cause and solidarity in the fight against the disease.

Blood donation
  use of antibody testing in,
        22, 45, 67, 93, 134, 145,
        162
  in U.K., 132
Blood products, imported, 143, 145
Brazil, 143
British Medical Research Council,
    93

Canada, 143
Caribbean countries, 42, 142, 146
Carriers, asymptomatic
  challenge to public health of, 19
  immunological parameters of, 47
Centers for Disease Control (U.S.),
        9, 21, 41, 42, 43, 57, 75,
        89, 113, 156, 157, 158
Central African Republic, 143
Children, 78, 96, 121
  right to attend school, 4, 19
Clinical trials, 50, 59, 90-91
Colorado
  antibody testing in, 26-27
  legislation in, 26-28
  management of AIDS epidemic in,
        23-28
  reporting requirements in, 26-27
Conferences, international, 42-43,
        145
Confidentiality, 18, 25, 30-31, 70,
        96, 136 (see also Medical
        records; Reporting of
        infection)
Contact tracing, 22, 27, 32, 33,
        34, 100
Counseling services, 22
  in Colorado, 27
  in San Francisco, 83, 84, 85, 88
  in U.K., 93, 134
Czechoslovakia, 143

Denmark, 143

Edinburgh, Scotland, 59, 92, 132,
        135, 145
Educational campaigns, 3, 11,
        16-17, 21-22, 25, 68, 98,
        145-146
  in Australia, 44-45, 46
  directed at drug users, 2, 21,
        68, 101-102, 134
  directed at health care workers,
        78, 134
  directed at homosexuals, 16-17,
        84, 133, 134
  effect on sexual behavior, 16-17,
        32
  funding for, 59, 70, 102, 125,
        158
  inoffensive language in, 21, 31,

Educational campaigns (continued)
  inoffensive language in
        (continued) 125, 127, 128,
        133
  "Madison Avenue" approach to, 21,
        123, 124-125
  in newspapers, 133-134
  public service messages, 84, 123,
        133
  in San Francisco, 32, 86, 122-123
  for students, 11, 21, 133, 134
  in Sweden, 101-102
  on television, 22, 86, 112-123
  in third world countries, 155
  in U.K., 93, 124-125, 127,
        133-134, 137
Europe, 143, 144 (see also specific
        country)

Federal Republic of Germany, 8, 143
Fogarty International Center
        (U.S.), 38-39
France, 8, 92, 143

Gay Men's Health Crisis (New York),
        106-107, 109, 124

Haiti, 114-116, 143
Health care, equity of access to,
        77-78
Health care costs, 81, 150
  in the future, 150-151, 158
  higher costs for AIDS patients,
        79, 80
  lifetime estimates of, 156-157
  in San Francisco, 86-87, 89,
        156-157
  in U.S. in 1985-1986, 157-158
Health care financing, 66-67,
        149-154, 161-163
  establishment of funding pool, 23
  in New York State, 78-79, 80, 81
  and patient migration, 152
  by public sector, 4, 81, 92, 94,
        151-152, 160
  in third world countries, 155-156
  in U.K., 94, 136
  (see also Insurance, health)
Health care workers
  attitudes of, 78
  educational campaigns for, 78,
        134
  protection of, 94
  team approach to care by, 82, 83
  (see also Nurses; Physicians)
Hemophiliacs
  AIDS cases among
    in Japan, 143
    in U.S. vs. Europe, 144
  infected with AIDS virus
    in Hungary, 145

New York City (continued)
  AIDS cases in, 95
intravenous drug users in, 2, 3,
      22, 95
  management of AIDS epidemic in,
      95-96
New York State, 1-2, 75-76
  AIDS cases in, 1, 142
  AIDS centers in, 2, 79-80
  hospital admissions in, 81
  legislation in, 79-80, 159, 160
  management of epidemic in, 77-80
Nurses, 85, 88, 89

Outpatient services, 46-49, 82, 83,
      85, 88, 89-90, 92
  data collection through, 46
Outreach programs, 50, 86

Pediatric AIDS, see Children
Physicians, 85
  information dissemination by, 84
  legal responsibilities of, 100
Prisons, 136
Privacy, see Individual rights
Prostitutes, 16, 99
  seroprevalence rate among,
    in Africa, 8, 10
    in Europe, 8, 92
    in U.K., 92
    in U.S., 8
  virus transmission via, 8, 9, 10
Public Health Service (U.S.), 22,
      41, 43
Public policy
  coercive, 16, 17
  proactive vs. reactive, 3
Public-private partnership, 82, 87

Quarantine, 16, 25, 27-28, 70, 100,
      101, 136, 137, 146

Reporting of infection, 20, 30-31,
      135-136
  in Colorado, 26-27
  in San Francisco, 83
  in Sweden, 99-100
  in U.K., 34, 92-93, 135-136
Respect for persons,
  justifications for infringing
      upon, 29-30
Rwanda, 9, 41, 143

San Francisco
  AIDS cases in, among homosexuals,
      82, 87
  antibody testing in, 83, 85
  cost of care in, 89, 156-157
  counseling services in, 83, 84,
      85, 88

San Francisco (continued)
  educational campaigns in, 32, 86,
      122-123
  funding of services in, 84-85
  history of AIDS epidemic in,
      31-32
  legislation in, 33
  management of AIDS epidemic in,
      82-91
  number of AIDS cases in, 81, 87
  reporting requirements in, 83
  seroprevalence rate among
      homosexuals in, 32
San Francisco General Hospital, 80,
      82, 83, 84, 85, 87, 88, 89,
      116-117, 156, 157
Screening, see Antibody testing
Sexual behavior,
  effect of education on, 16-17, 32
  "safe," 31, 67, 86, 97, 109, 133,
      134, 161
Sexually Transmitted Disease
      Service (U.K.), 92, 136
Shanti Project (San Francisco), 49,
      83, 85, 86, 88, 89, 90, 94
South Africa, 143
Surveillance, international,
      142-145
  in third world countries, 155
Sweden
  antibody testing in, 100, 101,
      102
  educational campaigns in, 101-102
  legislation in, 70-71, 100-101
  management of epidemic in, 99-102
  reporting requirements in, 99-100
Switzerland, 143, 145
Sydney AIDS Clinic (Australia), 44,
      46-50

Tanzania, 119-120, 143
Terrence Higgins Trust (U.K.), 93,
      94, 124
Therapeutic agents, 18, 55-56,
      90-91
Third world countries, 55, 58-59,
      68
  AIDS intervention programs in,
      154-156
Tunisia, 143

Uganda, 110, 143
Union of Soviet Socialist
      Republics, 143
United Kingdom
  AIDS cases in, 131
  antibody testing in, 93, 134-135
  cost of care in, 137
  educational campaigns in, 93,
      124-125, 127, 133-134, 137

United Kingdom (continued)
  health care funding in, 94, 136
  legislation, 93-94
  management of AIDS epidemic in,
      91-94
  reporting requirements in, 34,
      92-93
  seroprevalence rate in general
      population, 132, 145

Vaccine, 18, 55, 56, 60, 68-70, 71
  testing of, 52-53, 57, 68-70
Volunteer services, 102
  in Australia, 46, 49
  in New York State, 80
  in San Francisco, 83, 85, 86, 89
  in U.K., 124

Ward 86 (San Francisco), 83, 88
Women
  AIDS cases among
    in New York City, 95

Women (continued)
  infected with AIDS virus
    in Africa, 144
    in U.K., 132
  (see also specific risk groups)
Women, pregnant
  infected with AIDS virus
    in Brussels, 11
    in Kenya, 10
    in New York City, 96
  screening of, 11
  (see also Human immunodeficiency
      virus, maternal trans-
      mission of)
World Health Organization, 43, 57,
      142, 143, 145, 154-155, 156

Yugoslavia, 143, 145

Zaire, 9, 41, 42, 119, 143